Encyclopedia of Thai Massage

A Complete Guide to Traditional Thai Massage Therapy and Acupressure

Piere

C. Pierce Salguero

author of A Thai Herbal

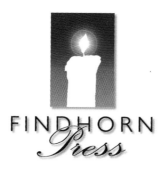

FINDHORN
Press

©C. Pierce Salguero 2004

First published by Findhorn Press in 2004
Reprinted 2005

ISBN 1-84409-029-9

Massage photography ©2003-2004
Christina M. Aucoin (christyaucoin@yahoo.com)

Back cover and page vi photograph of author by Dan Lopez ©2003 Daily Progress
(www.dailyprogress.com)

Other photography ©1997-2004
C. Pierce Salguero
(pierce@TaoMountain.org
www.TaoMountain.org)

Illustrations ©2001-2004 David O. Schuster
(www.DavidSchusterCreations.com)

Yoga Correlations ©2004 Kate Hallahan, R.Y.T.
(OmDaily@yahoo.com
www.TaoMountain.net/kate)

British Library Cataloguing-in-Publication Data.
A catalogue record for this book is available from the British Library.

Edited by Lynn Barton
Interior Design by C. Pierce Salguero and Thierry Bogliolo
Cover Design by Thierry Bogliolo

Printed and bound by WS Bookwell, Finland

Published by
Findhorn Press
305a The Park
Forres IV36 3TE
Scotland
tel 01309 690582
fax 01309 690036
info@findhornpress.com
www.findhornpress.com

Table of Contents

The Prayer of the Traditional Thai Healer v
About the Author vi
Preface vii

Part 1—Classic Thai Massage

Chapter 1: Introduction to the Tradition 3
    What is Thai Massage? 3
    History of Thai Massage 5
    Thai Massage Lineages 7
    Ethics in Thai Massage 8
    The Spirit of *Nuad Boran* 9
    Metta 11

Chapter 2: Before and After the Massage 13
    The Environment 13
    Interviewing the Client 14
    Working on Specific Conditions with Thai Massage 18
    After the Massage 19

Chapter 3: The Fundamentals of Thai Yoga Massage 21
    Overview of Thai Massage 21
    Basic Techniques 22
    The Pain Threshold 29
    Sen Lines in the Classic Routine 29
    Yoga and Breathing 35
    Rhythm of Thai Massage 36
    Body Mechanics 37
    Timeframes 37

Chapter 4: The Classic Thai Massage Routine 39
    Feet and Legs 39
    Hands and Arms 76
    Abdomen 87
    Yoga Stretches 95
    Back 117
    Head, Neck and Face 140

Chapter 5: Variations and Advanced Steps **147**
Variations for Side Position 148
Variations for Seated Position 156
Advanced Stretches 162
Walking Massage 171

Part 2—Thai Yoga Massage Therapy

Chapter 6: *Sen*, Thai Energy Lines **177**
Sen Lines 177
Northern and Southern Styles 189

Chapter 7: Thai Acupressure Therapy **191**
Acupressure Techniques 191
Hot and Cold Pressure 192
Acupressure Atlas 194

Chapter 8: Therapeutic Thai Massage **203**
Sen Line Diagnosis 203
Thai Massage, *Tridosha*, and the Four Elements 204
Sample Therapy Routines 204

Chapter 9: Thai Herbal Massage **234**
Thai Herbs and Massage 234
Herbal Compress Massage 234
Herbal Balms and Other Topical Application 237
Herbal Sauna or Steam Bath 238

Appendices

Endnotes and Sources 240
Anatomical Terms Used in this Book & Anatomy Charts 241
Where to study Thai Massage 244
Further Reading 247
Index 249

The Prayer of the Traditional Thai Healer

Om Namo Shivago Sirasa Ahang Karuniko Sapasatanang
Osata Tipamantang Papaso Suriyajantang
Komarapato Pagasesi Wantami Bandito
Sumetaso A-Loka Sumanahomi

Piyo-Tewa Manusanang Piyo-Proma Namutamo
Piyo-Naka Supananang Pinisriyong Namamihang
Namoputaya Navon-Navean Nasatit-Nasatean
A-Himama Navean-Nave Napitang-Vean Naveanmahako
A-Himama Piyongmama Namoputaya

Na-A Nava Loka Payati Winasanti

(Original Pali version)

We invite the spirit of our founder,
the Father Doctor "Shivago," who taught us through his saintly life.
Please bring to us knowledge of nature, and show us the true medicine in the universe.
Through this prayer, we request your help, that through our hands,
you will bring wholeness and health to the body of our client.

The god of healing dwells in the heavens high while mankind remains in the world below.
In the name of the founder, may the heavens be reflected in the earth,
so that this healing medicine may encircle the world.

We pray for the one whom we touch,
that they will be happy and that any illness will be released from them.

(trans. Chongkol Setthakorn)

Homage to you, Shivago, who established the rules and precepts.
I pray that kindness, wealth, medicine—everything comes to you.
I pray to you who brings light to everyone just as the sun and moon do,
who has perfect wisdom and who knows everything.

We honor you who are without defilement,
who are near to Enlightenment, having entered the stream three times.
We come to honor you. Honor to you. Honor to the Buddha.

I pray that with your help all sickness and disease
will be released from those whom I touch.

(trans. Ananda Apfelbaum)

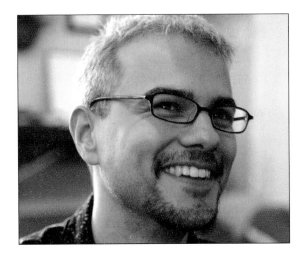

About the Author

Pierce is an accredited teacher of traditional Thai massage and herbal medicine, and is a member of the Shivagakomarpaj lineage, the Association of Northern Thai Medicine, the American Herbalists Guild, and the Associated Bodywork and Massage Professionals. His organization, the Tao Mountain School of Traditional Thai Massage and Herbal Medicine, is one of the top schools of Thai massage in the U.S., and maintains one of the most popular on-line sources of information on Thai healing traditions.

Pierce has degrees in Anthropology and East Asian Studies from the University of Virginia. From 1997 to 2001, he studied Thai massage and traditional herbalism under Lek Chaiya, Baan Nit, the Shivagakomarpaj Traditional Medicine Hospital, and other renowned schools in Chiang Mai, Thailand. He taught courses on traditional massage and herbal medicine at the Traditional Medicine Hospital in Chiang Mai, and from his home in a nearby village.

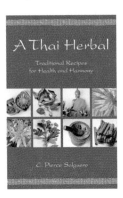

In September of 2001, Pierce moved to Charlottesville, Virginia, and founded the Tao Mountain School, which offers Basic, Advanced, and Teacher Training courses in the Shivago lineage of Thai massage. He is the author of *A Thai Herbal: Traditional Recipes for Health and Harmony*, the only English-language guide to the practice of Thai herbal medicine. (Also available from Findhorn Press.)

Preface

This is a comprehensive book explaining in detail the history, cultural context, and practice of the Thai art known as *nuad boran,* or *nuad paan bulan*. In English, this form of massage has been alternately called Thai yoga massage, Thai massage, and Thai yoga therapy. All of these terms (and several others) are used interchangeably to refer to the same style of bodywork which has been practiced in Thailand for hundreds—if not thousands—of years.

The manipulation of the body with intent to heal is a practice probably as old as the human body itself. The instinct to press one's head when it aches or to rub a sore calf muscle are precursors to this healing technique. What is impressive is the degree to which this natural instinct for healing touch has historically been developed and systematized in Asia while it has largely remained dormant in many Western cultures.

The great ancient civilizations of China and India developed complex medical traditions involving holistic approaches to total health of mind, body, and spirit. As these countries spread their spheres of influence through trade and religion, they exerted an enormous influence on the surrounding countries, including Siam, ancient Thailand, one land where these practices intersected, intermingled, and developed into a vibrant healing tradition. Long preserved in Thailand's Buddhist temples, which served as community centers and cultural libraries, the ancient wisdom was transmitted from teacher to student through oral tradition, resulting in the fascinating amalgam of mythology, medicine and spirituality that is today's *nuad boran*.

This book will cover many basic aspects of this massage, based on my experience as a student and a teacher in Thailand's finest massage training centers. There are several well-known bilingual schools in Thailand that cater to the Western tourist, presenting *nuad boran* in a digestible, step-by-step format useful for gleaning a basic knowledge of technique. I attended and later taught at such an institution, the Shivagakomarpaj Traditional Medicine Hospital of Chiang Mai, in northern Thailand.

The oral tradition is still honored in Thailand to this day, and most massage school teachers operate by verbally explaining and physically demonstrating each movement while their students listen and watch. Even in the massage schools that offer textbooks for their courses, the books are seldom more than a series of crude drawings. To this day, there has not been very much written on the subject of *nuad boran* theory either by Thais or by Western practitioners, and a systematic explanation of Thai medical theory is hard to come by. True to the Eastern tradition, Thai teachers are much less likely to give direct answers to theoretical questions, and will expect the students instead to learn these answers through their own diligence, practice, and patience.

The structured lessons at the hospital were invaluable as a base of knowledge for further practice. In my own experience, however, it was the contradictory and unstructured sessions with traditional practitioners outside of a formal institutional setting that elevated this technical knowledge to the realm of art. I learned that these masters had internalized their art so deeply that rote learning had given way entirely to the spirit. It was watching the graceful dances of these teachers that instilled in me an everlasting respect and love for their priceless cultural heritage.

I should say at the outset that any of these teachers would say it is impossible to learn from a book without hands-on guidance, and I would agree. Despite my best intentions to convey this information in its original format, as it is taught in Thailand, the reader must realize that learning any massage from a book is a vastly different experience than actual experience with a traditional teacher. This is especially true with healing techniques from the East, where teaching styles vary widely from the methods of our own culture. Far from the Western linear scientific approach to learning, students in Eastern countries absorb information from their teachers in a more formless manner, more often guided by intuition and creativity rather than memorization and systematic analysis.

It is in this creative spirit that many Western practitioners go on to combine *nuad boran* techniques with a wide range of other healing arts and other related fields from East and West (including Yoga Therapy, Swedish Massage, Reiki, Shiatsu, and other types of bodywork). In this book, on the contrary, I will allow the Thai tradition to stand on its own merits, as it is currently being taught in Thailand, in order to convey to the reader the depth and totality of this art. I feel that, in this modern day and age, it is of vital importance for us to conscientiously preserve and transmit ancient knowledge in its traditional format. I have brought to this book a discussion of proper alignment and safety from my practice of yoga, and a bit of modern anatomy, but other than these few points, I have endeavored to present this material as it was taught to me in Thailand, and as I saw it being practiced.

This book is an offering to my teachers, and to the lineage to which we belong. Despite the difficulty of spoken communication, my teachers taught me much with their hands, with gestures, and with endless patience and smiles. To Mama Lek, Pramost, Daeng, Wasan, Sutat, Pikun, Sasitorn, Song, Mama Nit, and to all my teachers, whether they taught me for months or hours, I gratefully dedicate this book.

C. Pierce Salguero
Nov. 21, 2003

Part 1
Classic Thai Massage

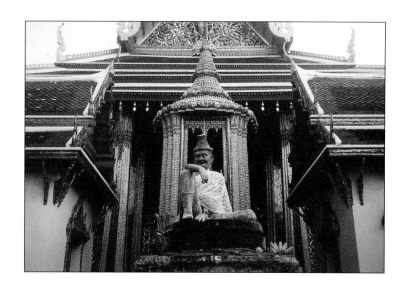

Chapter 1

Introduction to the Tradition

What is Thai Massage?

Thai massage, Thai yoga massage, Thai yoga therapy, *nuad boran*, *nuad paan bulan*, and *nuat thai*, are all names for a traditional healing modality which has been practiced in Thailand for centuries. Based on Ayurvedic medicine and yoga, this art form has been handed down through an unbroken chain of masters for centuries, and is practiced today across Thailand. Thai massage is becoming increasingly popular in the West, and is among the fastest growing massage modalities in the U.S. *Massage Magazine*, *Yoga Journal*, and other industry-leading consumer and professional magazines have frequently featured Thai massage in their pages.

A complete Thai massage incorporates a traditional combination of acupressure, energy meridian work, and yoga-like stretching. Thai massage is different from many Western forms of massage in that there is no oil used, the therapist uses a mattress on the floor (instead of a massage table), and that the client remains completely clothed throughout the session. It is so different from what we typically mean by "massage" that it is often instead described as having someone "do yoga to you." In fact, in Thailand, Thai massage has sometimes been called "yoga for lazy people"!

Thai massage is the perfect complement to any exercise routine and is suitable for clients of all ages and abilities. The classic Thai massage routine can be varied to suit a wide range of physical needs, and can be used as a form of physical therapy to aid in the increase of range of motion and muscular strength.

In modern Thailand, traditional massage is

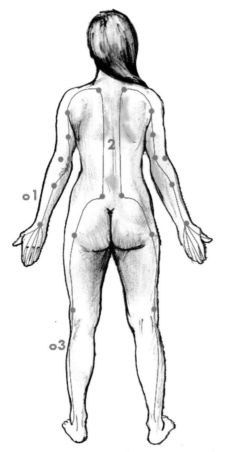

Some energy meridians and acupressure points on the back side of the body.

between specific points on the periphery of the body and the internal organs. Thus, even when treating a disease or injury associated with a particular part of the body, a therapist will typically work on acupressure points throughout. Linked through an intricate network of 72,000 energy meridians (*sen*), acupressure points stimulate and relax the patient's mind and body, promoting the natural healing processes.

These *sen* are of critical importance to Thai massage theory. In fact, in Thailand, Thai massage is considered to be energy–work rather than body-work. This is because the traditional therapist is guided not by anatomical structures or physiological principles, but by following the intricate network of energy meridians throughout the body. Even the yogic postures are considered primarily for their energetic effects, and only secondarily for their ability to improve flexibility and strength.

Although this art form was not developed with modern medical influence, we can clearly see that this massage routine has physiological benefits. Thai massage improves circulation, flexibility, and muscle tone. In many cases (such as over-worked muscles, fatigue, strains and sprains) properly administered Thai massage can take a vital role in repairing damaged tissue. This blend of acupressure and stretching is especially beneficial for those who find themselves stiff, sore, and tired from over-exertion in work or sports, or from arthritis or other disorders affecting mobility. Thai massage can often help these clients to recapture lost range of motion. By encouraging lymphatic function, this therapeutic deep tissue massage and stretching can also detoxify the body, heighten the immune system, and prevent disease and injury by promoting flexibility and supple joints and ligaments.

both a complex theoretical science, and an informal art form practiced by men and women throughout Thai society. On the one hand, Thai massage is a medical discipline, and is part of a four-year traditional medical university degree program. On the other hand, it is practiced in many villages by informally trained healers who have learned orally, without much theoretical background.

Thai massage is directly related to Ayurvedic principles originating in India, and is said to have arrived in Thailand along with Buddhism. Like other Asian massage techniques such as shiatsu and reflexology, Ayurvedic bodywork is a form of therapy based on the theory of the flow of energy

Of course, Thai massage therapists must recognize their limitations as well. In such cases as disease of the internal organs, chronic injuries, and degenerative conditions, the effects of the massage are difficult to gauge. As a holistic approach to healing, the most important function of *nuad boran* is to stimulate the body's natural healing process, and thus it can be an invaluable adjunct to any other form of treatment. It is unrealistic, however, to expect any massage to be a panacea, and even in Thailand, it is acknowledged that it is dangerous to rely on massage in lieu of proper medical attention. Although the benefits of Thai massage are wonderful indeed, under no circumstances should massage clients forgo consultation and treatment by a qualified medical professional.

The History of Thai Massage

Researchers have found indigenous Thai medicine to be an enigma, since the origins of this tradition are shrouded by centuries of secretive oral tradition. Viggo Brun and Trond Schumacher, in their analysis of traditional Thai medicine, point to the existence of two vastly different systems within Thailand, which they term the "Rural" and the "Royal" traditions.[1]

The rural traditions, according to Brun and Schumacher, are non-scholarly and rely on informal methods of education. These practices tend to vary considerably from village to village, and are transmitted largely through uneducated, local male practitioners who are closer to shamans, astrologers, and magicians than physicians. Their medical knowledge is handed down largely orally or through secret herbal manuscripts passed from teacher to pupil, and is usually not shared with outsiders, especially anthropologists or other Westerners attempting to study and understand their beliefs.[2] According to Brun and Schumacher, this form of medicine, utterly inaccessible to modern study, represents the indigenous Thai medical tradition, in existence prior to

the arrival of ideas from India and depending almost entirely on pre-Buddhist spiritual beliefs.

The Royal medical tradition, in contrast, developed at the royal court under direct influence from abroad. This royal tradition of Thai medicine is a complex system of intertwining cultural influences originating in India, China, the Muslim world, and the West, but the primary influence, at least as far as the theoretical body of knowledge is concerned, appears to have come from the Ayurvedic tradition from India.

Elements of Indian medicine are clearly evident in the earliest traditional Thai medical texts, but as these written records are certainly far more recent than the arrival of Buddhism in Thailand, they do not directly indicate when these ideas arrived or by what means. Somchintana Ratarasarn cites evidence that by A.D. 1600 the Royal medical tradition was well established in the capital. Even so, these records do not demonstrate at what point these ideas arrived in Thailand. The Thais date the introduction of Buddhism to Thailand to the reign of King Asoka (c. third century B.C.). The question as to whether elements of traditional Thai medicine arrived that early, with the introduction of Buddhism, or at a later date, remains unanswered.

The written record of the art of massage in Thailand dates to the same period. Massage is mentioned in seventeenth century palm-leaf medical scriptures written in Pali, the classical language of Theravada Buddhism. Writes Harald Brust:

These old texts seem to have been very important and were accorded respect similar to that bestowed on Buddhist scriptures. With the destruction of the old royal capital, Ayutthia, by Burmese invaders in 1767, most old texts were destroyed and are, sadly, gone forever. Only fragments survived and these were utilized in 1823 by

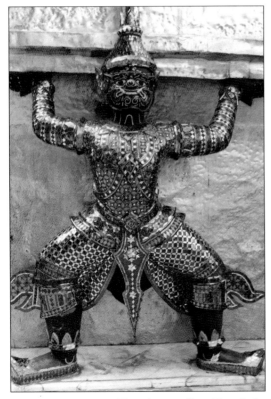

Temple guardian, Bangkok.

one looks at these diagrams with a Western concept of anatomy in mind, they appear to be quite strange at best, the reason being that anatomy did not play a role in ancient Thai massage. They are only a schematic device to show the pattern of invisible energy lines and acupressure points—and their influence on the body and its functioning.[4]

The tablets and statues at Wat Po show the high degree to which herbal and massage therapy had been codified and systematized in nineteenth–century Thailand. The correlation between the tablets and yoga shows that Indian ideas were deemed central to Thailand's royal medical tradition from at least around at the time of the construction of the temple. Also the inclusion of Ayurvedic diagnostic techniques and systems of classification, along with 1100 Ayurvedic recipes in Wat Po's herbal manuscripts from the nineteenth century show that Thai herbalists also saw Ayurvedic concepts to be central to their practice—at least in theory. But by the time of these inscriptions, Thai massage and traditional medicine seem to have taken their current forms.

King Rama III as the basis for the famous epigraphs at [Wat Po] in Bangkok. The fragments were collected and compared and then carved in stone and placed into the walls of the temple.[3]

The Wat Po diagrams are still a major source of technical information for therapists and scholars of *nuad boran*. These ancient diagrams describe a complex system of energy meridians and acupressure points, two ancient healing concepts which originated in India's Ayurvedic medicine. Harald Brust describes these diagrams thus:

These graven texts are still a rich source—and the only source—for anyone interested in exploring the theoretical background of Thai massage. Altogether there are 60 figures, 30 depicting the front of the body and 30 the back. On the figures therapy-points are shown along with the various energy lines called *sen* in Thai; these lines form the primary theoretical basis of Thai massage. If

The question remains: when did these Ayurvedic ideas arrive in Thailand? Based on my own research, my suspicion is that Indian and Thai medicine parted ways considerably earlier than the production of the Wat Po stone tablets. This would allow for either the complete integration of hatha yoga principles into an indigenous Thai massage, or else the development of an entirely new medical discipline, neither of which could probably have occurred only in the last few centuries. I hope to publish evidence for this speculation in an upcoming work.

What is clear, I believe, is that—regardless of the ultimate dating of its arrival in Thailand—the Indian medical system has for at least 500 years been used as an explanatory model by the Thais, has served as the core theory around which other indigenous ideas have been organized or explained, and has contributed greatly to several important Thai medical practices. Therefore, at least a cursory glance at the Indian traditions is unavoidable in any work on Thai massage traditions.

That being said, it is also clear that the Indian and the Thai practices parted ways many centuries ago, and that the two disciplines of Thai massage and yoga are not interchangeable. Thai beliefs, meridian charts, and massage techniques differ markedly from Indian Ayurvedic traditions, and can not be understood without looking at them on their own terms. This is what is attempted in this book, and while I will refer occasionally to parallels between the Thai and other traditions, it is always for point of comparison. In all cases, I give priority to the Thai tradition.

Thai Massage Lineages

Since its construction in the nineteenth century, the Wat Po temple in Bangkok, historically the center of the Royal Tradition of Thai medicine, has retained its importance as a medical facility. Housing the ancient stone tablets, the temple has long been a repository for healing techniques—something like a medical library of traditional herbalism and massage. At one time, massage was practiced at Wat Po primarily by the resident monks. Today, this is no longer the case as Wat Po is no longer a functioning monastery. However, to this day the temple is one of the most respected Thai massage and herbal medicine schools in the country, offering courses for Thais and Western tourists as well. This school has become the de facto headquarters of the Southern lineage, which is in fact known also as the "Wat Po Lineage."

The Shivagakomarpaj Institute, a traditional medicine hospital in Chiang Mai, northern Thailand, has also emerged recently as an important institute for traditional medical studies. This institute, affectionately known by its students as the "Traditional Medicine Hospital" or the "Old Medicine Hospital," emerged in the 1960s under the leadership of Ajahn Sintorn, who developed an innovative blend of the royal massage with indigenous influences from the Hill-Tribe regions surrounding Chiang Mai. The hospital offers courses to Western tourists, and serves as the head of the Northern lineage (also referred to as the "Shivagakomarpaj lineage" after the hospital).

As in many Asian arts, lineage is considered an important element of Thai massage instruction, as an indication of authenticity and a mark of high quality. There are also a number of traditional regulations and a code of ethics for the lineage, and lineage membership is considered crucial in Thailand, as it indicates that the practitioner is a member of an authentic and established tradition of Thai massage.

These two schools, the Northern and the Southern lineages, represent slightly different styles of Thai massage, and are compared briefly in Chapter 6. Despite these differences, however, the two lineages are very compatible, and may even appear to be indistinguishable to the untrained. Moreover, many practitioners in Thailand do not strictly conform to the Northern or Southern style, often combining techniques from many different traditions, including Burmese, Chinese, and Hill-Tribe massage.

Generally speaking, the two main lineages predominate, but influences and methods vary from village to village, special techniques are treasured from family to family, and styles vary from individual to individual, such that very distinct styles of massage co-exist side by side. Many of these informally-trained village practitioners exhibit a unique blend of royal and rural tradition, and are truly living examples of the very unique and colorful healing arts of Thailand. (For more information on these local practices, see the third book in this series, *The Spiritual Healing of Traditional Thailand.*)

Ethics in Thai Massage

The most basic ethical code observed traditionally in Thailand, regardless of lineage, is the Five Precepts of Buddhism, which are said to be basic rules laid down by the Buddha to encourage harmony among men. These principles are followed by Buddhists worldwide, and are translatable roughly as:

- Refrain from killing
- Refrain from stealing
- Refrain from dishonesty
- Refrain from drugs and alcohol
- Refrain from sexual misconduct

Buddhist culture traditionally emphasizes humility, honesty and compassion, and encourages the devout to practice these virtues in everyday life and livelihood. The practitioner of *nuad boran* is no exception to this rule.

In addition to classic Buddhist guidelines, the traditional Thai massage therapist abides by a separate code of ethics for the healer, taught in most of Thailand's massage schools on the very first day. This moral code is designed to protect the integrity of the tradition and to protect the client from unscrupulous therapists. These rules of conduct, as taught by the Traditional Medicine Hospital, are as follows:

1. Study diligently the techniques and the practice of the massage.
2. Do not practice in a public place or in a place otherwise unsuitable for massage.
3. Charge a fair price.
4. Do not take clients from another practitioner.
5. Do not boast about your knowledge.

6. Ask advice and listen to people who are more knowledgeable than you.
7. Bring a good reputation to the tradition of *nuad boran*.
8. Do not give certification in Thai massage to a person who is not qualified.
9. Give thanks to the Father Doctor before and after massage.

Despite the existence of this code of ethics, however, in more recent times, *nuad boran* has been somewhat tarnished by its association with the sex industry. In the last four decades of the twentieth century, particularly during the Vietnam War era, Thai massage became almost synonymous with prostitution. Countless massage clinics—particularly in Bangkok and Patthaya—served merely as fronts for brothels. The damage done to the tradition and the reputation of *nuad boran* during this time has carried over to the present day, and many still associate Thai massage with steamy Bangkok alleyways and illicit sex.

In the twenty-first century, however, this picture is far from the truth. While there remains in Thailand an illegal sex industry hiding behind many facades, most massage clinics today practice a legitimate, serious, traditional healing art which is an important continuation of ancient medical and spiritual knowledge into modern times. This is particularly true in Chiang Mai, which has long retained its well-deserved reputation as the most important center of traditional medicine schools in the country.

Attempts have been made in the last decades to develop a centralized organization on the national level in order to control the education and licensing of practitioners. Up until now, any traditional massage existing in Thailand could typically be given the label *nuad boran*. One of the goals of centralization is to standardize the practice and teaching of Thai massage to more accurately reflect the theoretical foundations of the royal tradition.

As already mentioned, part of the colorful diversity of traditional Thai medicine is the fact that there are so many different regional and cultural influences. While a national committee may do wonders in terms of quality-control and safety, it will have to tread lightly and carefully when it encounters and attempts to codify such diverse and mutually contradictory traditions as currently exist in Thailand. The unfortunate outcome of this process will be the loss of a large part of the informal beliefs and practices of the rural traditions.

Be that as it may, nationalization has already gone a long way towards restoring the legitimacy of the massage industry, and has done wonders to revive the respect due to these institutes of medical knowledge.

The Spirit of *Nuad Boran*

Thailand is an extremely devout country, where the most casual observer can readily see a deep and extensive Buddhist tradition influencing everyday lives. Buddhism and medicine have always been intimately interlinked in Thailand. In fact, it was the monasteries that carried herbal knowledge, Ayurvedic theory, and hatha yoga to Thailand from India in the first place. In addition to Wat Po, monasteries throughout Thailand continue to be important medical resources. In major urban centers, the monastic schools continue to produce many of the most educated individuals in a given city, and doctors are often present among the ranks of a monastery.

In rural Thailand, where formal education is more difficult to come by, charismatic monks are central in the practice of rural medicine, and still serve as modern-day shamans, offering healing amulets, magical protection charms, incantations, and exorcisms for the devout. While these practices may hearken back to pre-Buddhist times,

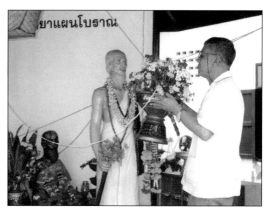

Ajahn Sintorn leads *wai khru* ceremony at the Traditional Medicine Hospital, Chiang Mai.

the imagery of the rites of rural medicine are Buddhist, the language of the incantations is often riddled with Buddhist phrases, and the location of the shamanic healings are usually community temples, indicating that Buddhist symbols play an important role.

At the center of the Thai healer's spiritual practice is Jivaka Komarabaccha (pronounced in Thailand as "Shivago Komarpaj") who is recognized as the progenitor of the traditional medical system. Shivago appears to have been a historical person. Buddhist historian Kenneth Zysk recounts the story of his early life, as told in the Pali scriptures:[5]

Salavati, a courtesan of Rajagaha, [gave] birth to a son who was then given to a slave woman, who placed him in a winnowing basket, which was thrown on a rubbish heap.... The infant is taken and raised by the king's son Abhaya.... The boy is given the name Jivaka because he was "alive" (from the root jiv, to live), and because a prince cared for him he is called Komarabhacca (nourished by a prince). Jivaka, as he approached the age at which he must seek his own livelihood, decided to learn the medical craft. Hearing about a world-famous physician in Taxila, he traveled to that city, famous for education, to apprentice with the eminent doctor. After seven years of medical study, he took a practical examination that tested his knowledge of medicinal herbs, passed with extraordinary success, and, with the blessings of his mentor, went off to practice medicine. [5]

Shivago is a minor figure in Buddhist scripture, but this story appears in various forms in Pali, Sanskrit, Chinese, and Tibetan translations. All versions of the scriptures agree that Shivago later became a Buddhist convert, the physician to the monastic order, and that at one point even treated the Buddha himself for an imbalanced *dosha* (Ayurvedic constitution).

Throughout the Buddhist world, Shivago has largely been forgotten, but in Thailand, this man has been elevated to the level of a deity. Shivago is believed by most Thai healers to be the ultimate source of Thai traditional medicine, and the inventor of the practices of Thai herbalism, massage, and acupressure. During my own research in Thailand, without exception, every healer I visited possessed a statue of the Father Doctor, seated or standing on the altar alongside the Buddha, in recognition of his position as the practitioner's primary *ajahn* (teacher or guru). This was the case equally for unlicensed, unofficial practitioners of hereditary forms of rural medicine and for formally trained practitioners and teachers of the royal tradition.

Shivago's statue is also placed in prominent locations in many monasteries and temples, including Thailand's national temple, Wat Phra Kaew, in Bangkok. (See photograph on the first page of this chapter.) A typical healer prays to Shivago for help in healing work, and patients often pray for a cure. Shivago is said to benevolently intercede on a patient's behalf, and is also said to transmit healing "through" the hands of the traditional Thai healer, who is seen as a conduit for this energy.

While most massage therapists put stock in the knowledge they possess and the techniques they perform, they put much more faith in the ability of the Father Doctor to guide their hands during the massage. Healers kneel at their clients' feet with folded hands and closed eyes and pray to Shivago for guidance in order to prepare themselves before each massage. Most practitioners feel themselves to be channels for the healing energy of the Father Doctor rather than healers in their own right. For the true master, every movement of the massage is an exercise in meditation and piety.

Many traditional massage schools teach as their first lesson the prayer to Shivago which appears at the beginning of this book. This chant to Shivago is recited in the Pali language, the traditional language of Theravada Buddhism, and is reproduced here as it appears in the student manual of the Traditional Medicine Hospital's basic massage course. The first English version, while not a precise translation, captures the essence of the prayer. This version, based on a translation by Chongkol Setthakorn for the Traditional Medicine Hospital, is also used at my schools in the U.S. The second English translation, from a recent translation by Ananda Apfelbaum, is a closer rendition of the original Pali text.[6]

In most Thai schools, this prayer (or a version of it) is chanted or sung every day in a ceremony known as *wai khru,* or "saluting the teacher." In the Traditional Medicine Hospital of Chiang Mai, where I first attended classes, it was chanted twice a day by the entire hospital staff, teachers, and students. Even at this, the most prestigious secular Thai massage and herbalism facility in the country (unaffiliated with any monastery), Shivago's ceremony is quite elaborate, incorporating Buddhist and pre-Buddhist rites, and reaffirming the central role of Buddhist faith and shamanic lore in the practice of Thai medicine.

In fact, one of the main teachings of the royal tradition is that religious practice is one of the major disciplines of Thai medicine, alongside herbalism and massage. The "Three Branches of Thai Medicine," as they are referred to, are represented in the architecture of the hospital itself, which houses a massage school and clinic in the West wing, an herbal dispensary in the East wing, and a pagoda containing the main shrine to the Buddha and Shivago in-between the two. The very placement of the shrine at the mid-point of the complex points to a self-consciousness about the centrality of Buddhist religion in the practice of traditional medicine. (For more on this topic, see my book *The Spiritual Healing of Traditional Thailand.*)

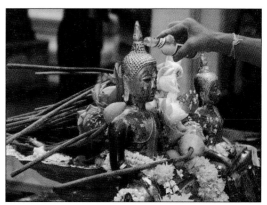

Anointing the Buddha altar with oil and flowers, Bangkok.

Another example of the spiritual nature of the practice is apparent in the various initiation ceremonies conducted by Thailand's massage schools. Many schools stand by a timeless tradition of initiation before the teaching may be imparted. Some of my Chiang Mai teachers asked me to bring nine fresh lotus flowers and nine sticks of incense (or another suitable offering) to perform a ceremony at their altar—which included images of Buddha and Shivago—before being accepted as a student. Equally noteworthy are the graduation ceremonies, such as the Traditional Medicine Hospital's farewell ritual which includes chanting, consecration of diplomas, and a binding of the students' wrists with sacred thread.

Metta

Most of the spiritual side of Thai massage is difficult for the Westerner to truly understand due to the language and cultural barriers that exist for the average tourist. Moreover, Thai massage schools for tourists are unfortunately not noted for their theoretical or spiritual teachings. To be fair, however, some of the most important practices in this art form are impossible to explain or learn verbally.

The true practice of the art of healing—be it *nuad boran* or any other type of medicine—is in the compassionate intent of the healer. The spiritual practices associated with Thai medicine, specifically the acts of piety and prayer, are Buddhist methods of building humility, awareness, and concentration in the healer and are designed to bring the practitioner to a deeper level of awareness of himself and the client. This compassionate state of mind is called *metta*, usually translated as "loving kindness."

Although the practice of Thai massage is always taught in a Buddhist context, the religious practices peculiar to that country need not deter beginning students from other cultures from studying this art form. Although I find the rich history and cultural heritage of the Buddhist Thai masters fascinating, I believe that both the massage and the cultivation of *metta* are fully compatible with any spiritual tradition. The most important lesson Thai Buddhism has to offer us is that it is universally desirable to make a sincere attempt to live honestly, humbly, and compassionately. Any spiritual practice that emphasizes these virtues will benefit the practice of a healing tradition by developing the intent to heal through touch.

Metta, coupled with proper understanding of technique, will in most cases guide the healer in performing the steps correctly, with the correct amount of intensity, and these actions will always be positive and helpful. However, if the mind is wandering or otherwise engaged, if the attention is not given to the client, or the compassionate intent to do good is absent, the massage will be nothing more than a series of empty physical movements. While these motions may have some benefit on their own, what benefit they have increases multiple times when the touch is infused with the will to heal.

It is for this reason more than any other that the Thai massage therapist begins his or her massage with a prayer to Shivago. In our Western context, a prayer, a short chant, or any other way of taking a moment to center ourselves, clear our minds, and focus on our clients, will work wonders for our practice and for our clients' well-being.

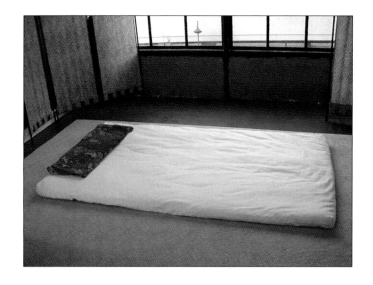

Chapter 2
Before and After the Massage

The Environment

Although the environment is often not given much thought in massage clinics in Thailand, it is a vital factor in the comfort of the client and of utmost importance to the Western practitioner. In Thailand, often massages are given in someone's living room with the television blaring, radio crackling, and people shuffling in and out. In many massage clinics, therapists gossip and lean over their clients to discuss their personal lives in loud voices, laughing and talking as much as massaging. This is because Thais consider massage to be a very commonplace and social facet of life, like going to the hairdresser in our own culture.

In our own society, massage is a unique and private experience, and practitioners must take care to ensure that their clients feel comfortable and relaxed throughout the appoint-

ment. For this reason, the environment is a vital consideration. Safety, clean work space, uninterrupted peaceful atmosphere, soothing lighting, and neat appearance are all vital to the Western massage clinic. Other considerations vital to the proper practice of Thai massage include:

Mattress: Use a thin mattress on the floor, a shiatsu mat, or Thai massage mat instead of a table. (See photo above.) A good Thai massage mat will usually be a pressed foam slab with a removable washable cover. This material is ideal because it is thin, supportive, and light.

Props: Keep plenty of pillows of different sizes handy to prop up different body parts throughout the massage. Blocks used for yoga practice also make great supports. In the winter, keep a blanket or sheet nearby to cover the parts of the body not being

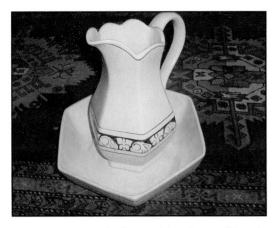

Basin for washing feet and hands

worked with, particularly when using herbal compresses. You may wish to keep a chair or ceiling rope in the work space for back-walking maneuvers (see Chapter 5).

Clothing: Thai massage is always performed fully clothed. Proper attire for the client and practitioner should include light, flexible clothing such as that used for yoga class. Clean clothing for the client should be kept in stock, in case the client comes unprepared.

Some other optional considerations to enhance the client's experience are listed below:

Aromatherapy: You may want to use scents to enhance the work space. Thai massage therapists often use Tiger Balm™ or other heating liniments after the massage in order to soothe muscles that have been working hard. If you use these or any aromatherapy products, always check with the client, and take care with stronger scents, as clients may find these intrusive.

Music: I do not like to use music with Thai massage because I feel that the rhythm of the music interferes with the natural rhythm of breath and movement that develops in silence. You may want to use soothing

non–rhythmic sounds such as recordings of rain, or a bubbling fountain if it helps a client to relax and enjoy the massage. Again, check with the client first.

Washing: In Thailand, it is common practice for the practitioner and client to wash hands and feet before and after each massage. Basins and soap are kept nearby for this purpose. In the West, hand-washing and proper care of bedding are recognized as key components in halting the spread of infectious diseases, and are an integral part of any massage clinic's safety regimen. For a touch of authenticity, you may wish to provide an attractive basin with soap and water and a towel for your client.

Interviewing the Client

It is vital to interview the client before each massage. It is important to be aware of each client's symptoms and limitations, and of any possible contraindications. Even a familiar client may present different symptoms or concerns during different sessions. It is important to get as complete an assessment of the client's total health condition as possible, as well as to discuss specific trouble areas before beginning the massage. On a practical note, detailed intake forms and client release forms are also required by most liability insurance companies.

On the next pages, you will find a sample intake questionnaire and release form from my own practice. You can photocopy these pages, or use them as a basis to write your own forms. The following are some general considerations to look for when conducting client interviews. (The answers to these questions will help you to determine the type of massage you will give each client.)

Client's age: You will have special considerations for very old and very young clients. Very young clients, such as infants, do not

Client Profile Form

Name: Age:

Telephone: or Email:

When and how do you prefer to be contacted?

What is (are) your primary complaint(s) or symptom(s)?

What is (are) your secondary complaint(s) or symptom(s)?

What is the history of these complaints?

Do you have, or have you had, any of the following (check all that apply):

___ high blood pressure   ___ high stress
___ low blood pressure   ___ nervousness/anxiety
___ high cholesterol   ___ diabetes
___ heart/circulatory disease   ___ frequent headaches
___ organ disease   ___ fatigue/weakness
___ chronic indigestion   ___ hormone imbalance
___ peptic ulcer   ___ irregular menstruation
___ chronic constipation   ___ cancer
___ irritable bowel   ___ other: _____

If you have a history of health problems of any kind, or if you are
currently on any medications, please elaborate:

Are you now, or could you be, pregnant? Please explain:

Please describe your eating habits:

Please describe your caffeine/nicotine/alcohol/drug intake:

Please describe your exercise habits:

Please include any additional information you feel would be helpful on reverse.

Massage Liability Release Form

You are about to become a client of _____ for the purpose of Thai massage and/or Thai herbal massage.

My certification to practice this art form is available for your inspection upon request.

Thai massage is not intended to cure, diagnose, or treat any medical conditions, and should not replace treatment or consultation with a qualified physician or therapist.

On rare occasions, clients may have adverse reactions to Thai massage. The symptoms may include headache, dizziness, muscle soreness, slight bruising, allergic reaction to herbal products, among others. If hot herbs are being used, there is the chance of slight burning. You are in complete control of the massage, and if you feel any of these symptoms at any time, please inform me so that I can correct the situation or discontinue the massage. By signing this release, you agree not to hold me liable for any adverse effects of any treatments given to you. *For your safety, please be sure to fill out my Client Profile form accurately.*

Thai massage is an intimate artform which requires the close contact of client and practitioner. I respect your privacy completely, and remind you that you remain in complete control of the massage at all times. If you feel uncomfortable at any time, for any reason, please inform me immediately, so I may take direct action to remedy the situation or discontinue the massage, whichever you prefer.

Your massage will be conducted in utmost confidentiality. Your personal information delivered during massage or on my Client Profile Form will not be shared with anyone for any reason.

_____ Please initial here, if you are receiving this massage in your home, to certify that you have requested this service.

By signing this form, you acknowledge that you have read and agree to the above.

Name:_____   Date:_____

Contact Information:_____

Date	Comments

require aggressive acupressure or deep yogic stretching. The younger the individual, the more naturally flexible they will be. Babies can benefit from light joint mobilization, gentle squeezing of the limbs, and superficial rubbing of the meridians. Children by age 8 or 10 can begin to perform yoga poses. Older clients will usually be restricted in their movements, particularly in the more advanced stretches. Elderly individuals usually can not stand deep presses or acupressure. They will, however, benefit greatly from the hot herbal compress massage discussed in Chapter 9.

Flexibility of joints & muscles: In clients of all ages, you will have special considerations for varying levels of flexibility. Most of the photos in Chapters 4 and 5 represent the ideal posture for the client. However, some alternative postures are show throughout the book for clients who are not as flexible (or those that are super flexible and need more of a challenge). Always keep in mind the alignment of the ideal posture, and help your client to work towards this goal. In time, you, and they, will see an increase in their flexibility.

Chronic injuries, pains, or problems on any part of the body: Massage steps that may aggravate existing injuries should be strictly avoided.

Back pain or inflexibility: You may want to avoid many of the back stretches in Chapter 4. When you are working on your client's back, he or she may be more comfortable in the side position presented in Chapter 5.

Heart or circulation problems: You may want to avoid steps which place the legs over the head, as well as all "blood stops."

Stress, Anxiety: You may wish to perform the massage at a slightly slower pace, with more of a relaxing intent.

Low energy conditions: You may wish to perform the massage at a slightly faster pace, with more of an energizing intent.

Food intake: Determine if the client has eaten recently. Clients should not eat three hours prior to a massage. If they have, be sure to skip the abdominal massage. You may have to omit some (or all) of the yoga stretches.

Menstruation: Due to abdominal distention and sensitivity, menstruating women should not receive direct pressure to this region unless the therapist is trained in this specialty.

Pregnancy: Under no circumstances should pregnant women receive Thai massage or acupressure from a therapist who is not trained in this particular specialty.

During the interview, the practitioner should also take into consideration the client's body size and shape in order to predetermine any additional props or equipment that will be needed. For instance, a small practitioner delivering a massage to a very large client, or a large practitioner delivering a massage to a small client, will present unique problems. In Thailand, very small Thai practitioners massage even the largest foreign tourists with little difficulty. Many massage steps give the therapist leverage through the skillful use of body weight and principles of physics, enabling him or her to handle even the largest clients. But this takes time and practice to perfect. When faced with any doubt as to your ability to perform specific massage steps, difficult steps should simply be avoided.

Under all circumstances, the practitioner should use his or her judgment when delivering a Thai massage. A very vigorous massage, *nuad boran* is best suited for healthy, active clients with minor ailments such as sore muscles or stress. Although Thai massage is used as rehabilitative therapy in Thailand, this should always be left to professionals trained in this specialty. Some rehabilitative considerations are presented in Part 2 of this book, but hands-on education is indispensible.

Working on Specific Conditions with Thai Massage

While performing a therapeutic Thai routine, you will run across specific conditions which will affect your choices during the massage. Different clients will present different abilities and challenges for you as a therapist. The object when working with any type of limitation is to keep in mind the ideal posture, and to aim for this with your client. You will need to keep their movements within their range of ability, while always encouraging them to expand their boundaries. Clients who receive regular massage usually find their range of motion increasing and symptoms such as pain and stiffness lessening, and often many chronic and acute diseases and disorders can be improved or healed.

The following are some considerations for working on specific conditions with Thai massage. In all cases, remember to use common sense, client feedback, and *metta* as your guides. More detailed therapeutic information is presented in Part 2 of this book. Hot compresses used throughout the massage will usually greatly increase the client's flexibility and dramatically lessen any of the following symptoms, in many cases enabling the client to receive a full session. (See Chapter 9 for more details on herbal compresses.)

Arthritis (or other chronic joint stiffness): This client will obviously need special care for most of the classic routine steps. However, yogic stretching is extremely effective in loosening joints and muscles, and can

be very beneficial for this type of disorder. Take clients to their limit gradually, slowly increasing intensity. Do not over-tax the joints. If the client experiences pain, ease off immediately.

Chronic Pain or Fibromyalgia: Many of the more advanced stretches in this book will be contraindicated. Only stretch the client within his or her limitations.

Back, Hip, or Sacroiliac Pain: Concentrate on steps which involve loosening the hamstrings and psoas. Do not over-exert the client, and be sure to skip the advanced yoga stretches.

Lower Gastrointestinal Disorder: This client will benefit from all forward bends and spinal twists, which will help to expel gas and promote digestion and excretion. Be careful with direct abdominal pressure.

Upper Gastrointestinal Disorder: These clients usually will not benefit from forward bends or spinal twists, which may aggravate acid reflux or ulcers. Do not apply direct abdominal pressure.

Respiratory Disease: Such clients may feel constricted or congested while lying down. You may wish to prop them up on a pillow. Perform seated variation from Chapter 5, focus on flushing the chest and abdominal region.

Menstruation, Post Partum, Obesity: Perform back massage from the side position in order not to put pressure on the abdomen.

Kidney Disease: Beware of stressing the lower back with intense stretches. Do not press directly on the kidneys (located along **back line 3**).

A more sophisticated approach to the treatment of specific conditions is to find the *sen* line associated with the symptoms, and to treat the *sen* accordingly. (Refer to Chapter 6 for more information on *sen* meridians.)

After the Massage

Sometimes, despite the best intentions of the practitioner, the client or the practitioner may experience an energy imbalance after a Thai massage. Often, this is accompanied by a feeling of being "wired," or hyperactive, with accompanying insomnia, or by a feeling of sluggishness, lethargy, and exhaustion. The causes of these energy imbalances can be numerous. If the client is feeling imbalanced, this could be due to an uneven massage. Perhaps both sides of the body were not treated equally, or the entire body was not massaged.

The imbalance may also, however, be caused by emotional release experienced during the massage, and thus represent a positive development. Many people respond quite dramatically to massage, especially if they are unaccustomed to being touched in such a manner. Reactions, such as tickling, tears, sexual arousal (including erections in men), emotional outbursts, and so forth, will occur, and the practitioner must be prepared to meet these situations as they arise. Patience and humor can go a long way under many circumstances. In many cases, the client may feel a bit embarrassed, but with a few kind words from the practitioner, will continue to enjoy the massage.

If the practitioner is feeling imbalanced or experiences strain, this may be due to overexertion or exhaustion or may be due to improper body mechanics. Thai massage techniques employ the principles of physics to ensure a smooth and easy massage every time. The practitioner should not feel drained by any motions, rather, both the client and practitioner should feel invigorated and relaxed by the sequence. Perhaps more practice is needed on particular steps in order to ensure smooth performance. If one is ever in doubt about a particular step, it is best to skip it.

Imbalances in the practitioner may also be caused, however, by a subconscious process of projection. Often, practitioners massaging clients with emotional outbursts will internalize the weight of these emotions, taking these emotions onto themselves. This must be avoided. The practitioner must learn to help clients dissipate their own negative energy; the practitioner must not contribute to the clients' negative energy or take it upon him/herself. The answer to this problem is the conscious intent of the practitioner and cultivation of metta. The practitioner must always envision him/herself imparting good energy and dissolving negativity during the massage. The practitioners will in time see that we all have an endless source of positive energy to give, and will avoid the temptation of falling victim to clients' negativities.

Sometimes the one who needs a massage the most is the one who is always giving them. The practitioner should never neglect him/herself. Under no circumstances should a practitioner give a massage while feeling unbalanced or negative, and sometimes receiving a massage helps to get the therapist back on track.

Guidelines for the Client
A Thai massage will rebalance the energy flow throughout the client's *sen* system. In order to protect the integrity of the energy work, Thai healers recommend not showering or eating for two hours after a treatment. Both of these activities interfere with the benefits of the energy work just completed. Other than this, let the client do whatever comes naturally, such as lying down, sleeping, etc. Providing space for clients to remain peaceful and comfortable after the massage ensures that they do not hve to get up and move before they are ready.

Guidelines for the Practitioner

Energetic issues for the therapist are different than those for the client. In many cases, practitioners of massage take on negative energy from their clients, letting their own systems become imbalanced. In order to regulate excessive or depleted energy the recommendations for the therapist are almost the opposite of those for the client: shower, stretch, do some self-massage or yoga, etc. In any event, take a break from the massage area for at least 30 minutes to recharge your batteries before starting another massage.

Also, remember that long-term energy-workers frequently need to take a short vacation from their intense work in order to rest and realign. Meditation retreats, yoga, and receiving massage can be great ways for therapists to periodically work on themselves. A daily tai chi, qi gong, or yoga routine can help to keep the practitioner energized and balanced, to prepare for the day's massage, and to help correct any energy imbalances caused daily. This is also an area that can be directly enhanced by a strong, positive, spiritual practice. Spiritual practice can teach us a healthy approach to healing, and valuable tools for taking care of ourselves.

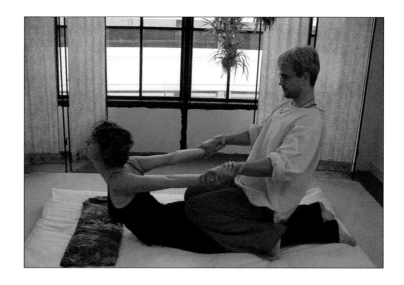

Chapter 3
The Fundamentals of Thai Yoga Massage

Overview of Thai Massage

Now that the preliminaries are out of the way with the previous chapter, we'll start in on Thai massage itself. In this chapter we will discuss the classic Thai massage routine. This is the type of massage you would give to the general population, a typical client with no special needs. Once you have mastered the classic routine (Chapter 4), you can progress to Chapter 5, where we will discuss variations and advanced moves, and then to Part 2 of the book, where we will focus on particular techniques and considerations for clients with particular types of disabilities and ailments.

When I first meet with clients who have never experienced Thai massage, and do not know what to expect, I typically tell them

that Thai massage is like "having someone do yoga to you." The massage is, in fact, truly not just a massage, but an integrated yoga class as well. An experienced therapist will assist clients to achieve yogic postures that they would not be able to experience on their own, and at the same time, will manipulate the muscles and tendons with the basic techniques we will discuss in a moment to assist with relaxation to facilitate the stretching process. In a nutshell, Thai massage typically consists of about half acupressure and half yoga stretches, and the practiced therapist will move back and forth between these two techniques with seamless fluidity.

The "classic" routine unfolds as follows: The therapist begins by warming up the clients body with light manipulation of the *sen* meridians, usually with thumb pressure.

This work will segway in most cases into a routine of gentle joint mobilization. The therapist will use his or her body to gently rotate the client's limbs, to lubricate the joints and to further prepare the client for the work ahead. When the preparation is deemed to be sufficient, the therapist will move into the third stage of the Thai massage, the yogic stretches, which is the climax of the routine. Once this stage has been completed, the therapist will cool down the client with gentle motions designed to soothe the hard-working muscles.

By following this sequence when giving a Thai massage, you will ensure that the massage has a flow and a rhythm that has been the hallmark of this unique art form for centuries. In addition to the preceding considerations, observe the Four Principles of Thai Massage listed on this page. These four principles each have their own rationale.

Basic Techniques

While the above summary may seem simple enough, there are many "hand techniques" employed by the Thai therapist throughout the course of a typical massage. These techniques range in pressure, and involve the precise use of body mechanics on the part of the practitioner. Beginning on the next page, these are discussed one by one. To ensure that you understand the jargon used later in this book, and particularly in Chapters 4 and 5, it would be best to familiarize yourself with these basic techniques before continuing on. Pay particular attention to the instructions in order to learn the principles of body mechanics from the very beginning. Establishing good habits early in your career as a Thai therapist will enable you to practice this art form over the long term with very little chance of hurting yourself.

The Four Principles of Thai Massage

Thai massage will always follow these four basic principles:

1. Always start from the extremities of the body (laterally), work towards the core of the body (medially), and then back to the extremities. The reasons for this are typically explained in terms of the flow of energy though the meridians, but may also be understood in terms of circulation of blood and lymph, assisting drainage of the extremities.

2. Always start from the bottom (the feet) and move towards the top (the head). The only exception to this rule is for the front of the torso, which is drained into the colon. The reasons for this principle have to do with the ancient Yogic notion that energy is purified as it moves up through the body. Most people will be familiar with the Indian *chakras*, which are the quintessential examples of this general rule.

3. Always perform meridian work first, then joint mobilization, then yogic stretching. This rule is simply so that clients are warmed up — physically and energetically — by the time they are expected to stretch their limbs.

4. Give a balanced massage. Steps you perform to one side, you should perform to the other. Remember that the entire body should be massaged — even if only a short massage is given — in order to keep the body's energies balanced. If you are just performing a foot massage, massage the hands too in order to bring balance to the body. Or, if you are giving a quick shoulder and neck rub, press a few acupressure points on the feet to even out the energy. The results of energy imbalance can leave your client feeling either wired or tired! (See Chapter 2.)

Palm Press

The palm press is the most basic technique in Thai massage. The most important factor in performing this technique correctly is that you must position your core (your waist and hips) directly over the client, so that your body weight is translated directly through the shoulders, elbows, and wrists. Your arms should be straight, to provide an uninterrupted flow of body weight. Place your palms so that the fingers point away from each other for a "but-

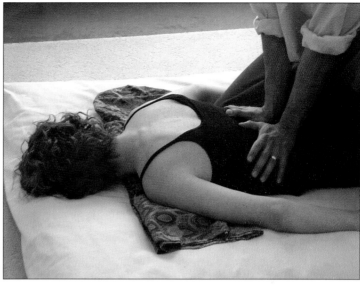

terfly palm press." Use gravity to apply the pressure, not upper body strength. Your palms should be spread widely so that your weight is distributed over the maximum surface area. Think of the way a cat "paws" at the carpet.

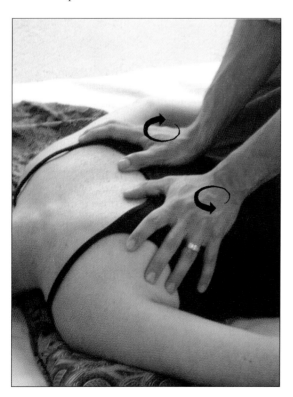

Palm Circles

This is a lighter touch than the palm press, although the principles are the same. Your palms are spread out, and your finger tips are engaged. Use your fingers and palms together in a gentle circular motion. Palm circles are used to stimulate areas that are potentially sensitive, such as the abdomen and the rib cage. You are not applying your full body weight in this move.

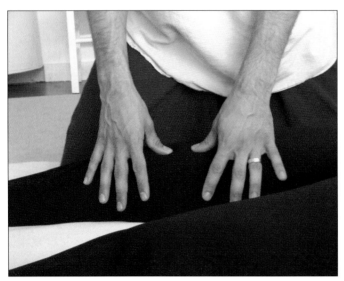

Correct

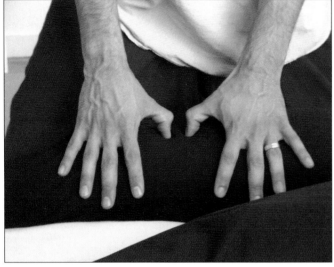

Incorrect

Thumb Press

The basic Thai massage method for applying acupressure, the thumb press, is used mainly on muscles and energy meridians. Never press directly on bone with a thumb press, and be sensitive to the client's threshold for pain. Thumb presses should be stimulating and strong, but not overwhelming.

The top photo shows a correct thumb press. Proper alignment of your body includes proper placement of your shoulders directly above your hands. Keeping your elbows and wrists straight, press with the ball of your thumb, arms straight, using your body weight to apply pressure.

The bottom photo shows an incorrect thumb press. Note that the bend in the thumbs causes the body weight to have to take a 90° turn at the thumb knuckles. This will inevitably lead to soreness, inflammation, and eventual tissue damage for the therapist. Note that the correct method involves keeping the thumbs straight and closely in to the palm of the hand. The pressure is always applied with the ball of the thumb, not the tip.

Not only are there physiological reasons why this proper alignment should be observed, but also energetic reasons. Proper alignment keeps your own energy flowing uninhibited through your hands.

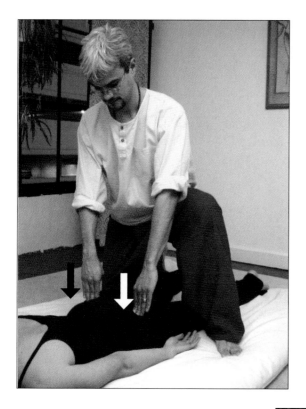

Finger Press

The finger press, or the "bladed hand" is used when thumb press does not provide proper leverage, or when trying to press a very thin area. Finger presses are used on the psoas, under the clavicles, and on the glutes. Finger presses are lighter than thumb presses, although not quite as light as the finger circles. Your body should be positioned so that this movement is natural, without strain on the back or arms. Again, your body weight is translated through straight arms, straight wrists, and straight fingers. This move utilizes only body weight, no arm strength.

Finger Circles

Finger circles are generally used over the sensitive parts of the body, for example on the temples, skull, sacrum, and sternum. The body weight is translated through straight arms and straight wrists, but avoid applying too much pressure. The finger circle is the lightest touch in Thai massage. Your body is positioned so that your core (your hips and waist) are positioned directly over the client. Your body weight is translated through straight arms, wrists, and fingers.

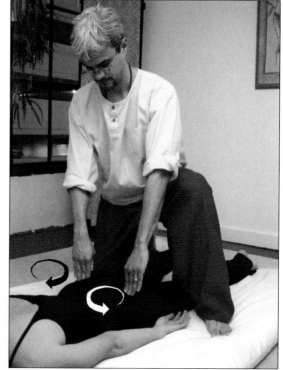

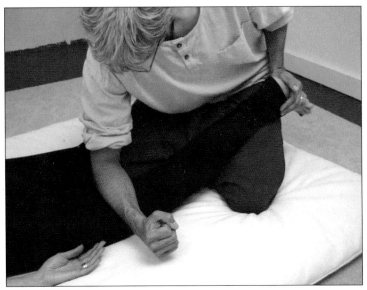

Forearm Roll

When you want to apply more pressure than you can with the palms, the forearm roll is the next option. Your body weight is translated through your shoulder to your bent elbow. Be sure to perform the roll with the part of the forearm closest to the elbow. If you use the wrist, you will put strain on the elbow joint itself. This move is used particularly on the backs of the legs, although you can try it in other positions on clients who enjoy more pressure.

Elbow Press

The elbow press is one of the most famous Thai massage techniques. The sharp point of the elbow makes it a useful tool to apply greater pressure to acupressure points with accuracy and force. The elbow is usually used on the hamstrings, glutes, feet, and other large muscles that are not as sensitive.

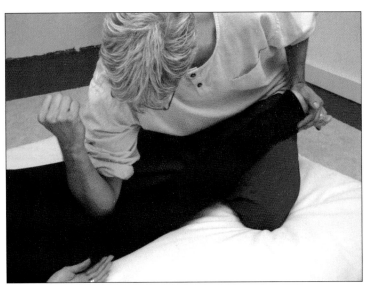

Beware of using your elbow on areas where it may cause pain or bruising. Proper alignment requires the same principles as the forearm roll. This time, however, the pressure is delivered through the tip of the elbow. Lean into your elbow to apply pressure, and slowly unbend your arm to remove the pressure. Be sure to always use your body weight, in order not to over-tax your upper body muscle strength.

Advanced Presses

The knee press, foot press, and heel press are used only in specific cases.

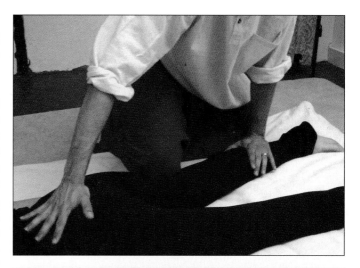

There are a few moves where these presses are used while you are seated so that you can apply pressure and preserve proper body mechanics. Such moves are possible to perform on most clients. Some moves, however, require you to stand or kneel over the client. Due to the intensity of this pressure, these techniques are usually best reserved for large, muscular clients with whom you has already established a relationship and who appreciate deep work.

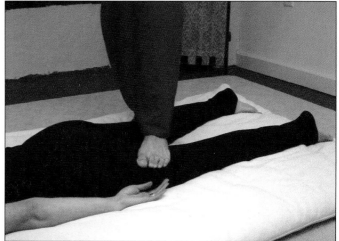

The foot press is discussed in more detail in Chapter 5, where walking on the client's back is introduced. You should be aware of safety considerations, especially with the foot presses, and avoid slipping or losing balance while employing these techniques. Use a nearby chair or a ceiling rope to help you to balance.

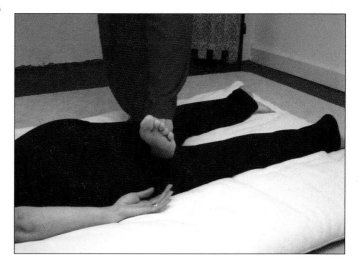

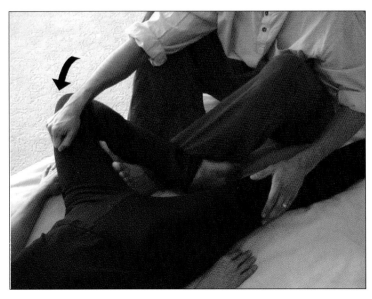

"Thai Fist"

The "Thai fist" is used to encourage circulation to muscles, and is a good "cool-down" technique for a muscle that has been working hard. Loosely cup your hand, and knock the client's muscle with your curled fingers. Keeping your hand loose will make a soft patting sound.

"Thai Chop"

The "Thai chop" is another cool-down move which is relaxing and remarkably soothing for worked muscles. The Thai chop seems easy, but is difficult to perform correctly. Spreading your fingers widely, press your finger tips firmly together while keeping the rest of your hand relaxed. Your palms should be cupped, lightly touching. Move your arms from the wrists, keeping your elbows outward and unmoving. Quickly but gently strike the client with your little finger, and allow the rest of your fingers to fall into place. The sound made by your fingers hitting together will be echoed by your cupped palms, and will result in a "clacking" sound. With practice, this sound will become very loud, although the client will not feel jarred. Move the Thai Chop around the muscle group to relax.

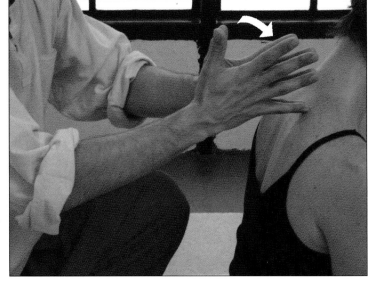

The Pain Threshold

Although Thai massage is a deep form of bodywork, the basic techniques introduced on the previous pages span a range of pressure, and not all Thai work needs to be deep. In general, Thais prefer deep, forceful presses and strong stretches. There often seems to be an attitude of "the more pain the better." However, this strategy will obviously not win over many clients in the West.

With time, you will learn to feel the client's needs with your hands as you work, and will naturally find the appropriate level of pressure for each individual. The important thing is to be aware of each client's pain threshold. If your client is interested in relaxation, try to avoid this threshold with a lighter touch. If your client likes to be challenged, however, you can take him or her to this threshold and slightly beyond. Controlled strong work will open the client's muscles, promote energy flow, and improve flexibility over time.

Sen Lines in the Classic Routine

The concept of invisible energy meridians coursing throughout the body is commonly used in the practice of most Asian medical traditions. Of these traditions, the energy meridians most commonly known in the West are those used in Chinese Medicine. As mentioned in Chapter 1, the Thai energy lines, or *sen* as they are called in Thai, are in fact more closely related to the *nadis* of the Indian traditions of yoga and Ayurveda.

The Spectrum of Pressure

Less Pressure ← → More Pressure

finger circle — thumb circle — palm circle — finger press — thumb press — palm press — forearm press — elbow press — knee press — foot press — heel press

It is said in the Thai tradition that there are 72,000 *sen* lines. (Some sources also mention 2700.) This should not, however, be taken literally. This number is a traditional Buddhist way of indicating an infinite amount, the point being that every cell in the body is linked to every other cell through this infinite and intricate mesh of energy. This energy is known as *prana* (Sanskrit), *chi* (Chinese), or *palang sak* (Thai). The pranic networks permeate the body of any living being, and vibrate in response to physiological, psychological, and spiritual experiences. This energy also emanates from the body, creating an electromagnetic field around the organism commonly known as an aura, or a "pranic sheath."

No one can name and diagram all of the body's infinite energy circuits. However, 10 main *sen* are commonly taught and used in Thailand's massage schools to treat the entire body. These 10 *sen* are the main conduits, the "highways" of energy in the body, off of which the rest of the *sen* branch.

The diagrams on the following pages show various parts of the body with the associated portions of the 10 main *sen* lines. (How these *sen* segments fit into the classic Thai routine is discussed in Chapter 4 at the appropriate step.) You will note in the following *sen* diagrams some red points along each line. These are important acupressure points which lie along each meridian. These will be covered in more detail in Chapter 7, when we discuss acupressure therapy. However, I present them now, as they may prove to be valuable landmarks which will help you to find the *sen* lines. In the context of a classic Thai massage, these acupressure points should be treated as any other point along the sen line. Simply run through the point with thumb presses as you move up the meridian. However, in the context of a therapeutic massage introduced in Part 2 of this book, you will be using these points to stimulate energy in particular areas of the body to treat a wide range of diseases and disorders.

Also note that in these charts the terminology commonly used for labeling the *sen* line

segments is introduced. The abbreviations *o* and *i* stand for *outer* and *inner* sen lines. Thus, line o1 refers to the first outer line. Note that there is an o1 in the arms and an o1 in the legs. These are not actually the same meridian. The abbreviation o1 in these cases means simply the first outer line of the arms and legs respectively. The terminology *o1, o2, o3*, etc., will be used as a shorthand throughout the rest of this book to refer to specific portions of the meridians we will encounter during the classic routine introduced in Chapter 4.

While anatomy is not usually a significant part of traditional training programs in Thai massage, for the purposes of conveying information in a concise and precise manner, I have used some basic anatomical terms throughout this book. For more information on anatomy, consult the anatomical charts and recommended reading at the end of this book.

Sen Segments in Head and Neck

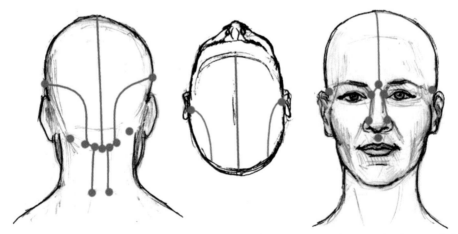

Two lines rise up along the neck vertebrae from C7 vertebra to the base of the skull. These become three lines, two of which round the head 2-3 inches behind the ear, and terminate at the temples. The third follows the midline of the head from the base of the skull, over the crown to the "third eye" notch, between the eyebrows. This line becomes two again, branching along the bridge of the nose to each of the nostrils.

Sen Segments in Legs

On the medial side of the leg, the first inner leg line (i1) runs from the front of the ankle, along the medial side of the tibia, through the medial side of the knee, along the medial side of the femur, and ends at the groin. The second inner leg line (i2) runs from the medial side of the ankle, along the medial side of the calf and thigh, and ends at the groin. The third inner leg line (i3) runs along the posterior side of the leg from the Achilles tendon, up the posterior side of the calf and hamstring, to end at the top of the femur.

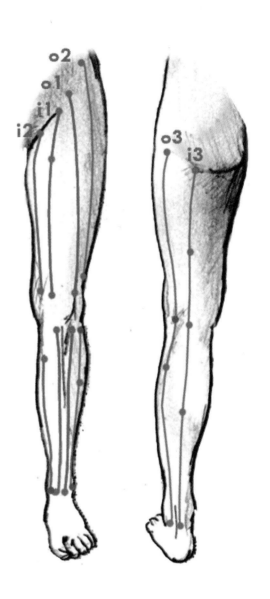

On the lateral side of the leg, the first outer leg line (o1) runs from the top of the ankle, along the lateral side of the inter-condylar eminence of the tibia, through the lateral side of the knee, along the lateral side of the femur, to end at the hip flexor. The second outer leg line (o2) runs from the outside of the ankle, up the lateral side of the calf, along the tensor fasciae latae, to end at the head of the femur. The third outer leg line (o3) begins between the ankle and Achilles tendon, up the outside of the calf, along the lateral side of the hamstring, to end at the head of the femur.

Note that all lines except i3 and o3 skip over the knee. It is believed that the lines travel through the joint itself, thus they are not worked on directly in this region. Because there is no bone on the back of the knee, the third inner and outer leg lines can be worked through the joint.

Different views of the leg are presented here and on the next page to give you the best possible understanding of the course of these lines.

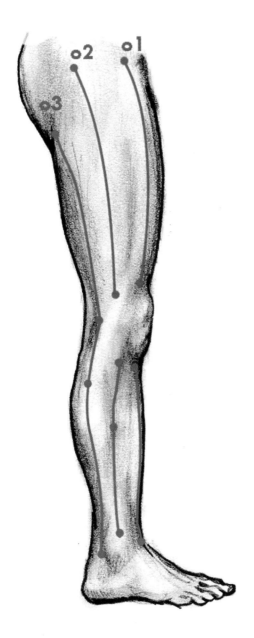

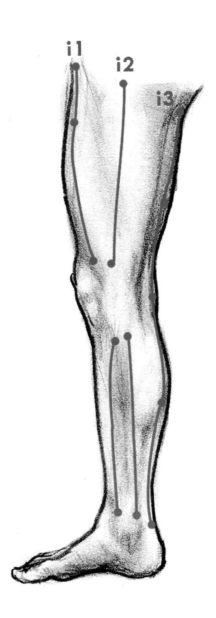

Lateral
Side

Medial
Side

Sen Segments in Arms

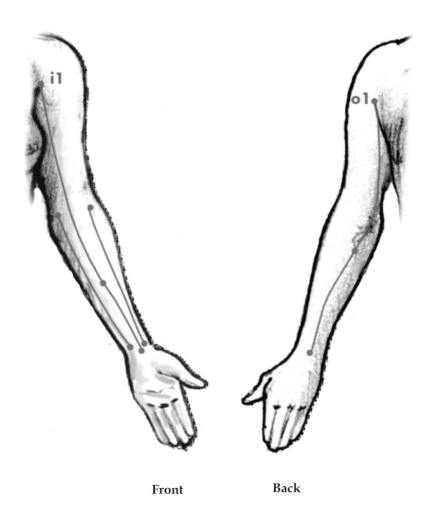

Front   Back

The outer arm line (o1) runs along the posterior side of the arm, beginning at the wrist joint. It runs in between the radius and the ulna, along the medial side of the humerus, and ends under the acromion process of the scapula. The inner arm line (i1) runs along the anterior side of the arm from the wrist joint, up the middle of the forearm, through the elbow, along the medial side of the humerus, and ends at the arm pit. Two branches of this line begin at the wrist and run along the medial side of the radius and ulna respectively, terminating in the elbow.

Sen Segments in the Back

The first back lines run from the sacroiliac joint, immediately alongside the spine, up to the C7 vertebra. Press in between each vertebra, particularly at the L1-2 and T4-5 junctions. Pressure should be applied in a medial direction (towards the spine). The second back lines run from the top of the iliac bone about a half inch laterally from the first back line. This line runs along the muscles to either side the spine. Pressure should be applied in a lateral direction (away from the spine). The third back lines run from the iliac crest along side the lumbar fascia and iliocostalis lumborum, to end above the shoulder blade. Pressure should be applied in a medial direction on the lower portion of these lines, but when at the scapula, press down and laterally into the rhomboids.

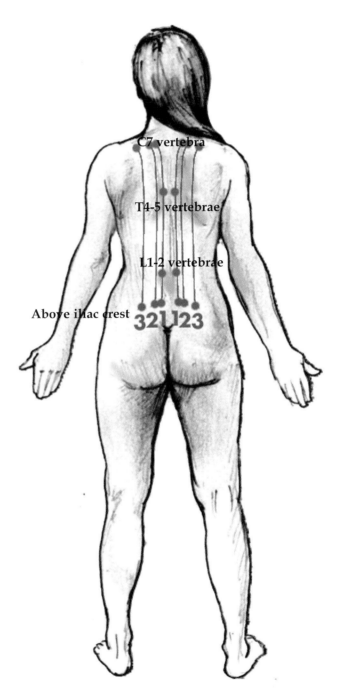

C7 vertebra

T4-5 vertebrae

L1-2 vertebrae

Above iliac crest   3 2 1 1 2 3

Yoga and Breathing

Yoga has been a part of Thai massage since the very earliest times. Although in India, the art of yoga developed into an individual spiritual practice, in Thailand, it is largely seen as a collective medical practice. Modern Thailand does not have a tradition of individually practiced yoga (except for what schools have recently come from India, mostly to meet the needs of tourists).

The fact is, however, most Thais will be familiar with some basic yogic principles. Most Thais are also familiar with the techniques of Thai massage, having grown up with these methods in their cities or villages. However, many Western clients will not be so familiar with either. For them, some explanation may be necessary before embarking on a Thai massage. Communication is your most important tool. Be sure that your clients are aware of what will transpire before you place them into some of the more advanced, and potentially scary, positions.

How intensive of a yoga workout is given will always depend on the ability level of the client as well as the goals of the massage. It is the therapist's duty to recognize the first hint of pain or uncomfortable pressure in a client and to adjust to this reality immediately. That being said, however, the experienced therapist will be able to determine the difference between true pain, which indicates danger, and the healthy feeling which comes from stretching and challenging the muscles.

The practitioner of Thai massage will have to work hard to develop the ability to "hear with the hands." A Thai massage is like a dialogue with the client's body, and the experienced therapist will be able to know the appropriate amount of pressure to use with each client. This is a sensitivity which takes a long time to develop, and until it does, a

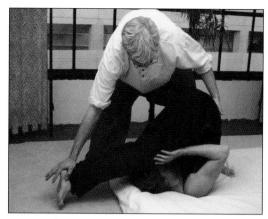

Breathing is especially important during the more intensive yogic stretches.

practitioner's best course of action is to hold back during a massage.

When first starting out, pay attention to the feeling of the client's limbs as you stretch them. If you are paying close attention, you will be able to feel the point at which the muscles are beginning to reach their maximum stretch. You should encourage the muscles to stretch, but not overdo this. Improperly administered Thai massage can and will cause muscle strain, pulled muscles, and other dangerous side-effects. I always recommend that my students take classes in yoga (particularly in an anatomically precise tradition such as Iyengar) so that they may experience first-hand the feeling of stretching, and can therefore become more empathetic Thai massage therapists. A yoga practice of your own can help you to better understand the physiology of stretching, and to recognize the experiences of your clients.

Once you become adept at finding the proper level of stretch, you can assist your clients to gain flexibility and joint mobility by helping them to achieve deeper and deeper stretches. The main mechanism for this progress is proper breathing. As with any yoga session, breathing is critical in Thai massage. The breath is a very useful aid in relaxing muscles. When putting clients into a stretch, it is always more beneficial for them if they can breathe deeply into the abdomen rather than hold their breath (which will probably be their first reaction). Deep breathing relaxes the lower abdomen, the iliopsoas muscle, the lower back, and the diaphragm, and greatly reduces tension throughout the entire body. Deep exhalation also detoxifies by releasing stagnant energy, gasses, and other waste materials broken up during a massage from the body.

It is not always easy for clients to remember to breathe, especially in deeper stretches. Work together with your clients. Begin by explaining the benefits of deep breathing, and then help them be aware of their breath throughout the massage.

Concentrate on the rhythm of the client's breathing during the massage, and set your pace by this. Bring the stretch deeper with the client's exhalation, and ease off a bit with each inhalation. The client establishes the pace; your job is to respond to this cadence. Soon, if you are lucky, you will find yourself moving and also breathing in harmony with your client's breathing without thinking. When you find yourself in this situation, locked into a beautiful dance of grace and breath with another individual, you will discover why this art form has been called a "moving meditation."

Rhythm of Thai Massage

Learning Thai massage can often feel like rote memorization at first. But, the sequence as it is presented in this book and as it is presented in Thailand's many massage schools, is a tried-and-true system of massage that has been perfected for centuries. These moves are ordered in this way not because of someone's whim, but because the steps work together in this particular way. Often, a stretch is followed by a counter-stretch which is designed to release the muscles previously worked. Usually, there are also energetic reasons for the order of the movements. Once you have read Chapter 6 and are more familiar with the energy meridians, you will discover why it is that certain steps are placed in a certain order.

In any event, it is also important to learn the Thai massage steps in the order they are presented here because it is crucial to develop a smooth sequence to provide a regular flow and rhythm, giving a more relaxing experience to the client, and avoiding redundancy. The steps here flow from one to the next seamlessly, and as the practitioner becomes increasingly familiar with the moves, he or she will find that they blend together into a routine (like a dance or a tai chi form) which is deeply satisfying to the practitioner. How are Thai massage therapists able to work for 8 hours straight giving one massage after another in Thailand's famous clinics? It is because their work itself is constantly regulating their energy, moving energy through their bodies in a way that sitting at a desk never could!

Some clients will choose Thai massage for the relaxation that it can bring. Others will prefer to be energized by the deep stretching and bodywork. Both these types of clients will enjoy Thai massage because it is a versatile art form. The same massage can serve to relax or invigorate a client, depending on the speed, duration, and intensity of the routine. For an invigorating massage, the movements should be shorter, faster, with more rigorous pressing. The Southern style of Thai massage in particular emphasizes quick, strong stretching movements. For a relaxing massage, the movements should be closer to Northern style: longer, slower, and more gentle.

In either case, it is the intent of the practitioner that truly determines the client's experience. Thought is a powerful force that leads

energy. Keeping the intent to impart soothing and relaxing vibrations to the client in
the foreground of the mind is enough to
make this a reality. Similarly, the intent to
impart energy and vitalization to the client is
enough to make it happen if one remains
mentally focused.

Body Mechanics

One of the most dangerous pitfalls that a Thai
massage practitioner can face is improper body
mechanics. In Thailand, typically small female
Thai practitioners are able to massage hulking
tourists seemingly effortlessly. With proper
body mechanics, therapists can give an effective massage to someone almost twice their size
or weight without feeling drained or exhaust-
ed. With improper body mechanics, however,
practitioners are in danger of injuring themselves and/or their client.

Back pain, repetitive stress injuries, joint pain,
and other injuries that plague many Western
massage therapists are not usually a problem
for Thai practitioners who use correct body
mechanics. Important principles of body
mechanics are discussed throughout
Chapter 4, but they can be recapped here
briefly as well:

1. Always keep your back straight.
2. Your strength comes from your legs and
hips, not your arms or back.
3. Translate body weight though straight
elbows, wrists, and fingers.
4. When you need increased leverage, bring
your center of gravity (your waist) up over
the client.

Understanding and using gravity, fulcrums
and other principles of physics which are
discussed throughout Chapter 4, the therapist will always deliver an effective massage
while preserving his or her own well-being.

Timeframes

In Thailand, the classic Thai massage lasts an
hour and a half. In most massage clinics, this
is the minimum time for a massage, and a
client can typically request a massage ranging up to 3 hours or more.

Westerners, accustomed to paying for a half
hour or, at the most, a 1 hour massage, will
initially need some explanation. As soon as
they receive their first Thai massage, however, they will see that this timeframe is in fact
a good minimum, leaving the therapist
enough leeway to cover the entire body
effectively.

My students usually react to the news that
they have to give a 1.5 hour massage with
fear, usually due to the thought, "How am I
going to fill up all of this time?" They are
soon surprised, however, by the fact that time
seems to fly when giving a Thai massage.
Especially while they are learning the routine, Thai therapists sometimes find that they
are rushing through their routine in order to
fit it all in to that length of time!

The following are some suggested routines
for Thai massage of varying lengths.

3 hour massage: For highly stressed or
lethargic individuals, or for those requiring
major therapy. Should not be given by inex-
perienced practitioners to avoid fatigue.
Perform all steps in Chapters 4 and 5, plus
herbal compresses.

2 hour massage: For stressed, fatigued, or ill
clients. Follow all steps in Chapters 4 and 5.
Or, perform a 1.5 hour classic massage routine, and add herbal compresses.

1.5 hour massage: The "classic routine." This
is the minimum duration for a massage at
most massage clinics in Thailand, and a good
duration for basic Thai massage. Perform all

steps in Chapter 4. Work in steps or variations from Chapter 5 as time allows. A good rule of thumb is to spend 50 minutes on the front side of the body, turn the client and work on the back sideof the body for 30 minutes, and finish with the head and neck for 10 minutes.

1 hour massage: A trial massage, to give the client a demo. Perform all steps in the classic routine (Chapter 4), skipping either Advanced Stretches or meridian work.

.5 hour massage: Perfect for chair massage. Massage head and shoulders, feet and hands. Use seated variations from Chapter 5. Remember to press acupressure points at the extremities in order to balance the energy throughout the body.

Recommended Frequency of Massage: Under normal circumstances, average clients looking for relaxation and invigoration should not get more than two massages a week, although daily massage is quite alright for short-term relief at particularly stressful times. Therapeutic massage clients should be seen according to the type of complaint. Acute injuries should be seen daily until the problem is relieved. Chronic cases should be seen on a weekly or—at maximum—a twice-weekly basis.

The reason that these recommendations are made is that there is such a thing as too much Thai massage. Clients who are constantly stimulated by deep Thai work over a long period of time can actually become depleted of energy, no matter how good the therapist is.

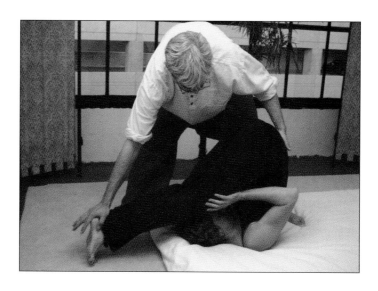

Chapter 4
The Classic Thai Massage Routine

This chapter will walk you through the 108 steps of a classic Thai massage routine in detail. The routine in this chapter is specific to the Northern Thai lineage, but is similar to the Thai massage you would receive across Thailand or from any Thai practitioner.

The steps outlined in this chapter are arranged in a specific order, based on the principles of energy work in the body. A Southern style massage would present these steps in a different way, however; each lineage has its own reasons for ordering steps, and these decisions are not arbitrary. Therefore, it is of utmost importance that you follow the steps as they are presented in this book. Once you are familiar with the energetic principles behind this routine, you can experiment with replacing some steps with others. However, this practice should be strictly

reserved for the advanced practitioner.

As stated in the previous chapter, this classic Thai massage routine is designed to impart a balancing and invigorating experience for the majority of your clientele. However, always be sure to work within the ability of each individual client, and to honor his or her needs and limitations.

For reasons of simplicity and clarity and because a female model representing the client appears in the photographs, the client is referred to throughout as *she* and *her*.

One last note: Be sure to completely read the previous chapters before diving in, as many additional points of safety and body mechanics, as well as terminology and theoretical concepts, are discussed earlier in this book.

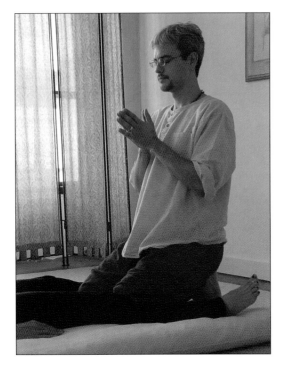

1. Opening Prayer

Every traditional Thai massage begins with a prayer to the Father Doctor Shivago, to request that the healing energies of the universe come through the therapist's hands in order to help the client.

This moment of silence is also a chance for you to center yourself, to forget about the busy day you may have been having up to this point, and to align your intentions as best you can with the needs of your client. Be sure to take this moment to ground yourself before you touch the client and "plug in" to her energy system. Your massage will be that much more effective and beneficial for those that you touch when you calm your mind, deepen your breathing, and cultivate *metta*. (See Chapter 1 for more details on the spirituality of Thai massage.)

ॐ Correlations with Yoga ॐ

Throughout this chapter, parallels between Thai massage and yoga therapy will be pointed out. The reader should note that the sections on yoga are not intended to be a comprehensive explanation of that art form. I highly recommend that my students participate in a yoga class (particularly one with a high degree of focus on proper alignment and anatomical principles such as Iyengar). However, this

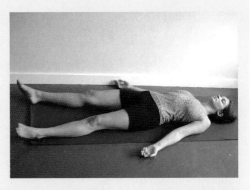

book is not intended to be an introduction to these postures, and injury can result from attempting some of these positions without guidance. I offer these correlations strictly as a point of comparison for those already familiar with the yoga tradition, and encourage those who wish to learn more to seek out a competent teacher.

The client's beginning position is known in yoga as *savasana*. This pose is for relaxation and inward reflection. Place the client's arms on either side of her torso, palms facing upward. Spread her legs apart 30° to 45°, and allow her feet to fall open naturally. Her shoulders should be even, and should fall down against the mat. The client should breathe naturally, into the abdomen, and allow her back muscles to release towards the floor.

Feet and Legs

2. Walking Palm Press
Northern lineage Thai massage starts at the lower part of the body and moves up because of the concept of the purification of energy as it rises through the body. (See Chapter 3 for more details.) Our first contact with the client, therefore, is with the soles of the feet.

In this step, keep your hands relaxed, like big cat paws, and evenly distribute your body weight through your hands. Keep your wrists directly under your shoulders, and your arms completely straight. Lean from side to side transferring your body weight. Your palms walk across the client's feet from the toes to the heels. Repeat a couple of times.

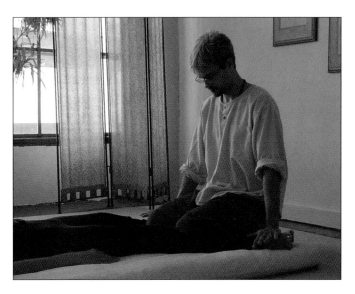

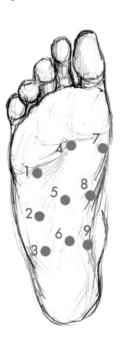
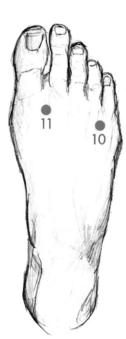

3. Thumb Press the Feet
There are six important acupressure points on the sole of each foot (1-6), and three along the arch (7-9). Starting with the points that are further to the lateral, or the outer, side of the body, and starting from the toe to heel, move your way across all nine points, pressing each several times with firm thumb presses. You can do two feet at the same time if you wish, or one at a time if you find this easier.

Then, turn the foot so that you can press the points on the top of the foot. Take the thumb and put it between the knuckles of the fourth and fifth toes. There should be a point (10) that is rather sensitive, and which sends a little "zing" through the foot. The second point (11) is the exact same place between the knuckles of the big toe and the second toe. Press each point a couple of times.

Note that while the sole and arch can take quite a bit of pressure, you do not need a lot of strength on the points on the top of the feet, as they are very sensitive. If the client experiences pain with a thumb press, small thumb circles would work on these points just as well.

4. Thumb Circles on Foot

Taking the left foot for a female client, or the right foot for a male, thumb circle the sole of the foot, drawing a line from each toe to the heel. You can do one toe at a time, or two together. Apply thumb presses to the points on the toes as shown in the diagram at right.

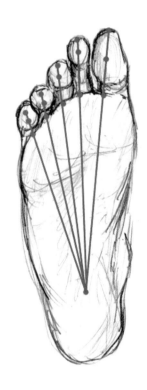

Next, start from the point right in front of the ankle (see red dot in photo below). From this point, follow the extensor digitorum tendons down to each toe with finger circles. Move down to the fifth toe first, stopping to thumb circle the knuckles. Repeat for each toe, moving from lateral to medial, from the pinky to the big toe.

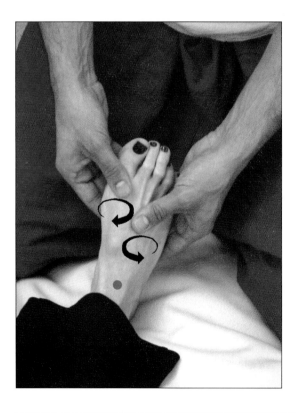

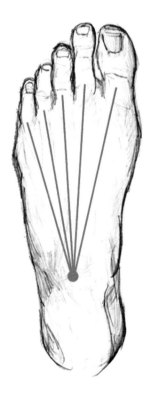

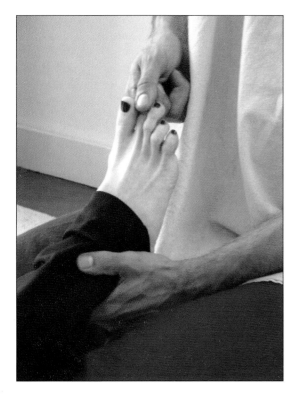

5. Pull Each Toe to Crack Knuckles

In Thailand, the Thai massage therapist is your chiropractor, and when you go for a Thai massage, the therapist makes a point of cracking all of the knuckles on the toes and fingers. It is your choice if you wish to do this as a Thai therapist. Contrary to popular myth, cracking your knuckles does not make your knuckles fat. The sound is just a part of the natural realignment of the bones. The gasses stuck between the bones release with a cracking sound as they are placed back into alignment.

Rotate each toe clockwise and counterclockwise five times in each direction to warm it up, and then, using a moderate amount of pressure, just straighten it out. There is no need to yank the toe hard, just give a little traction and if it needs realignment it will crack.

ॐ **Correlations with Yoga** ॐ

The foot series on the following pages relates to a group of yogic exercises for the joints known collectively in Sanskrit as *Pawanmuktasana*.

Therapeutic Benefit: These exercises are designed to improve the joints by encouraging movement and flexibility. They are used in particular to ward off or to treat arthritis, stiffness, and injury.

Contraindications: Caution is advised with clients who have pain in the feet or ankles, including arthritis, plantar fasciitis, or acute injury.

6. Twisting the Foot and Rotating the Ankle

The foot twist is shown in the top right and bottom left photos. First, support the heel with one hand and hook your other around the foot so your fingers touch the sole. In this position, by leaning back, you should be able to twist the foot to the outside. Keep in mind that we are never using muscle strength in Thai massage, but always body weight. Avoid "wringing out" the foot with your hands. With the correct hand hold, you simply lean back, and the foot twists without any effort on your part. When you switch the position of your hands as shown in the bottom left photo, the foot twists to the inside.

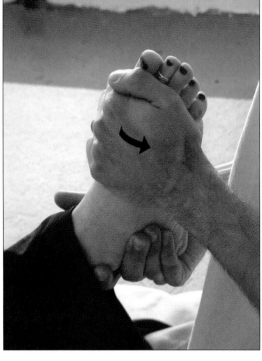

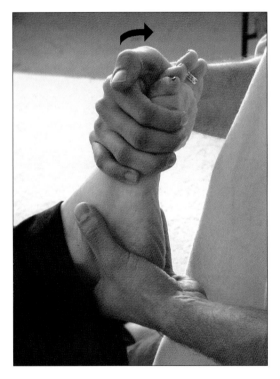

7. Ankle Rotation

The ankle rotation is shown in the photo in the bottom right. This is again not your arm muscles doing the work, but a gentle motion in your hips. Circle five times around in each direction–clockwise and counter–clockwise.

Repeat Steps 3-7 for the other foot

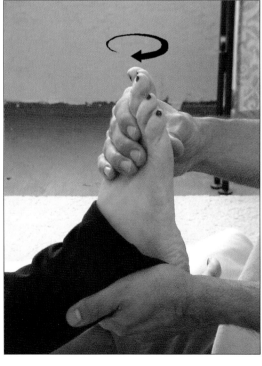

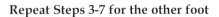

8. Stretching the Feet and Ankles

For the first stretch, place your hands on the top of the client's feet, aligning her ankles with her legs. Apply your body weight to bring the soles of her feet towards the floor. Do this three times.

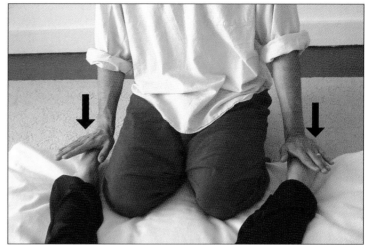

The second stretch brings the client's toes up toward her head, stretching out the sole of her foot. Be sure to properly align the foot so that the inner and outer arches are stretched evenly. Remember, this is a stretch for the feet and toes. The idea isn't to get under the toes and stretch the hamstrings, but to get over the toes and concentrate on the sole of the foot. Push the client's toes back and towards her head.

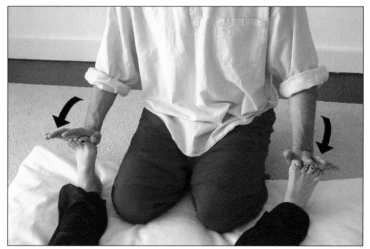

The last of these three stretches is to bring both the client's feet to the inside. Press down, with straight arms so that your body weight comes down on the tops of her feet, bringing the inner arches towards the mat.

Remember, different clients have different levels of flexibility, therefore how far you push or how much body weight you use in these moves will vary.

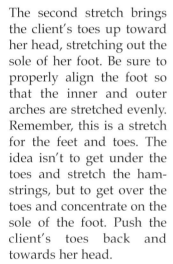

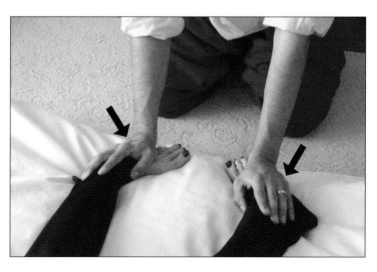

9. Palm Pressing Both Legs

At first, this looks like a repeat of Step 2, as you begin by palm pressing from the client's toes up the feet to the ankles. Be sure to do this with walking palm presses, leaning from side to side for best use of body mechanics. This time instead of going back down the feet, continue up to the knees, palm pressing the soft part of the calf without pressing directly on the shin bone. When you reach the knees, put your palms right over them, and gently rotate the kneecaps. Never apply body weight directly to the knees. Rotate them clockwise and counterclockwise, four to five times in each direction.

Continue with your walking palm presses up the client's legs until you reach the tops of the quadriceps muscles. For the upper legs, notice in the photo to the right that I have lifted myself up off my knees to bring my body weight over the client. This is to keep my back straight and let gravity do the work.

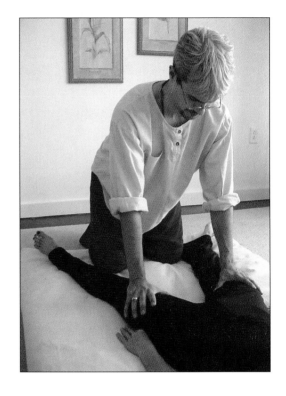

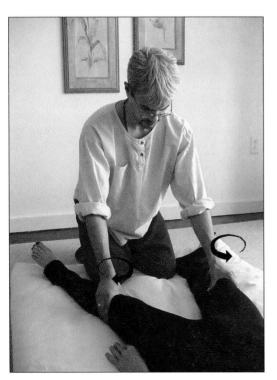

Stop right under the hip bone and then proceed back down. Move down the thigh with walking palm presses. Stop for palm circles at the knees, and then palm press back down the lower legs, through the ankles, and down to the toes.

Note that for these palm presses, when you are leaning from side to side you should be slightly rolling the client's legs to the outside because of the way your body weight comes down. On the thighs it is especially important to have the "cat paws" — wide-spread fingers and wide palm — in order to provide a large area for the distribution of your body weight. The reason is that the thigh is particularly vulnerable to having the muscle split over the bone. If you apply pressure straight down with the heel of your palm, it can be painful. So, always be sure to gently and evenly roll the muscle to the outside as you walk up the legs.

10. Stretch Inside of Leg

The next three steps will be a series which will appear again and again each time you work on energy meridians in a section of the body. For each of the four limbs and the back, you will always first stretch, then palm press, then thumb press, then palm press, then stretch. I call this the A-B-C-B-A pattern.

Begin with the right leg for men, or left leg for women. For the first step, position yourself so that your arms are straight out in front of you on the client's leg. Place one hand on her inner thigh, and one on her foot. Shifting your body weight forward, give her leg a gentle stretch to align it and lay out the inner leg meridians before you.

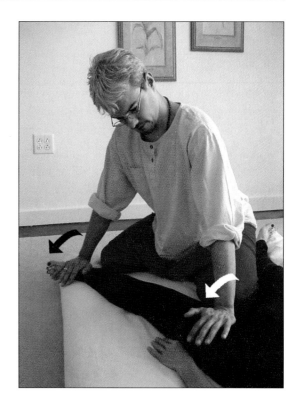

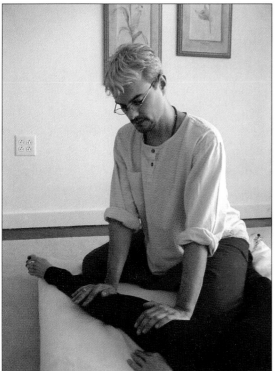

11. Palm Press Inside of Leg

Apply walking palm presses to the inside of the leg, as always beginning from the foot and moving up towards the inner thigh, and then back down again to the feet. Cover the entire inner thigh area with wide "cat paws." Skip over the knee to avoid pressing on the bone.

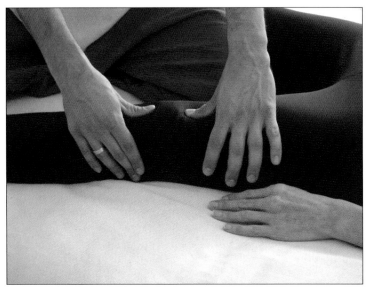

12. Thumb Press Inside *Sen* Lines of Leg

Following the guidelines in Chapter 3, apply thumb presses along the inner leg meridians i1 and i2. From this position, it is not advantageous to work on the line i3. We will leave this for when the client turns over onto her back.

Remember, work these meridians from the foot to the upper thigh and back down to the foot.

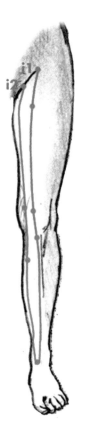

Finish by Repeating Palm Press and Stretch to Complete the A-B-C-B-A Pattern

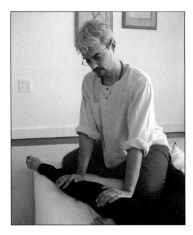
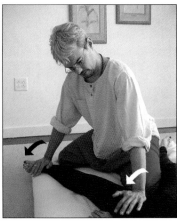

13. Stretch Outside of Same Leg

Having worked on the inner leg, move your stance to the outside of the client's same leg to work the outer meridians. Repeat the A-B-C-B-A pattern. Begin again with a stretch. Place one of your hands just under her hip bones in the soft part of the thigh, and your other hand on the top of her foot. Placing your hands in butterfly position, apply your body weight evenly into both your hands. Be sure that you are pressing the foot in toward the midline of the body to give a stretch across the outside of her leg.

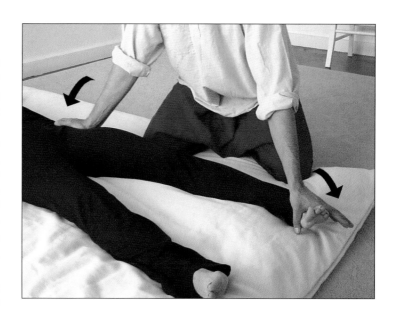

14. Palm Press Outside of Leg

Palm press, starting from the foot, moving up towards the hip, and then back down to the foot. Be sure not to press on bone, and to skip over the knee.

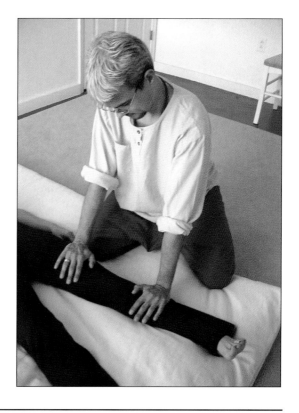

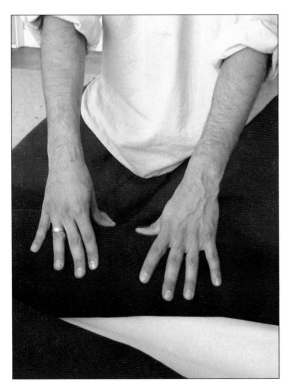

15. Thumb Press Outside *Sen* Lines of Leg

Following the guidelines in Chapter 3, apply thumb presses to outer leg *sen* o1, o2, and o3. Start at the ankle, proceed up the leg to the hip, and then back down again.

Finish by Repeating Palm Press & Stretch to Complete the A-B-C-B-A Pattern.

Then, Repeat Steps 10-15 for Other Leg

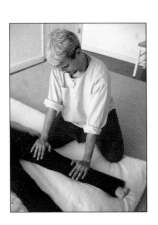

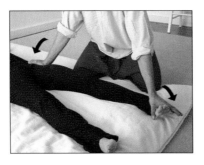

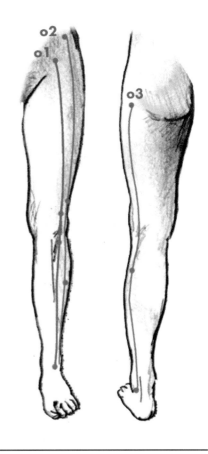

Alternate Position for Leg Lines

When you are more familiar with the meridians in the legs, you can use this alternate position to thumb press two at a time. In this position, press o1 first. Next, press o2 and i1 together. Next, press o3 and i2 together.

Don't forget to start at the ankle, and work up to the hip, and then back down again.

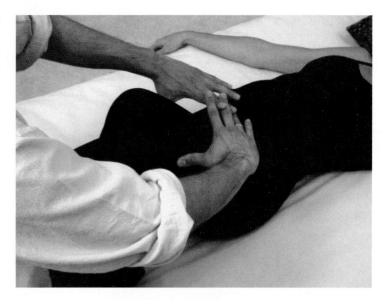

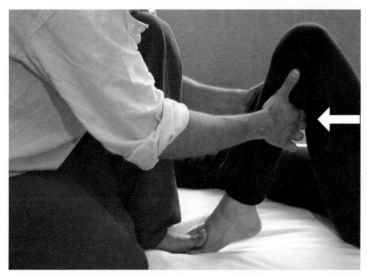

Next, pull along line i3, starting from the ankle, and moving up towards the knee. When you arrive at the calf muscle, pull towards you, lifting the client's heel as shown in the photo. Use your foot to keep her foot on the ground. Continue up i3 to the hip, and then work your way back down.

This alternate method will make your leg meridian routine quite a bit quicker; however, it should not be attempted until you are thoroughly familiar with the exact position of each *sen* line.

This routine can also be used in conjunction with the previously introduced routine in order to provide additional stimulus to the leg lines.

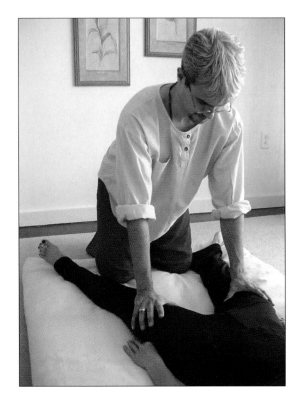

16. Finish the Leg Meridians with a Palm Press and "Blood Stop"

Step 16 is initially the same as Step 8. The palm press is both the warm-up and cool-down for the leg lines. Palm press the client's legs up to the knees, and palm circle the knees as before. Then, adjust your weight so that your center of gravity is over the client, your arms remaining perpendicular to the ground, and continue the palm presses up the quadriceps.

At this point, when your palms arrive at the top of the quads, place your hands directly over the spot on the leg where you would feel the femoral pulse. This point is along line i2, slightly below the groin, and to the inside of the femur (see photo below). With your hands in "butterfly" position, fingers spread out away from each other, apply your body weight to this point.

This move is called the "blood stop." Thai therapists use blood stops at the femoral artery to flush the energy system of the legs. Applying body weight to this point, the blood supply to the legs is lessened dramatically and the legs may begin to tingle. Hold this stop for 10 seconds, and then release.

As the blood rushes back into the legs, palm press the legs back down to the toes, bringing fresh blood to the furthest extremity. The client should feel a rush of warmth through her legs.

Be sure not to perform this or any blood stop on clients with circulatory or cardiac disorders, including, but not limited to hypertension, varicose veins, and heart disease.

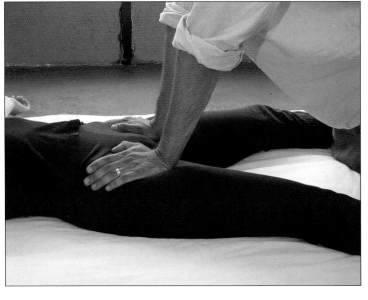

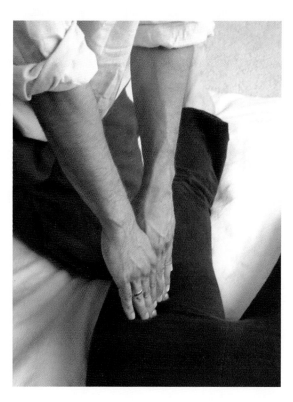

Advanced Variation for Femoral Blood Stop

This is an option which you may wish to perform in clients who enjoy deeper work.

In this step, a finger press is used on the blood stop point. This can be a sensitive area, so beware of applying too much pressure.

While you are here, you can also use the bladed hands in this position to press along the iliopsoas muscle in order to encourage it to relax.

Be sure to use discretion any time you employ this type of deep pressure.

Repeat on both sides.

17. Figure 4 Walking Palm Press

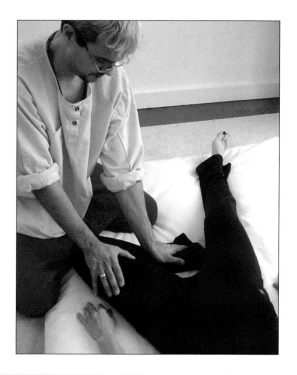

Start with the left leg for women or the right leg for men. Place the client's foot by her opposite knee to make a "figure 4." Put your hands in butterfly position, with your fingers facing away from each other, for a walking palm press on her bent leg. As always, your body weight is above the client. The palms come down on the soft parts of the legs, the inner thigh and calf muscle, not the shin bone.

Walk from the knee out to the hip and ankle, and then back to the knee. Apply more body weight to give a deeper stretch to the hip. Use only a little body weight at first, but gradually increase with each press until you reach your maximum.

18. Figure 4 Hip Stretch

This is the first of the series of joint mobilizations. From this step forward, proper breathing becomes essential for the client. One of the key physiological and energetic points to keep in mind is that the speed, rhythm, and deepness of the breath regulates the relaxation of the muscles and the body. If your client is holding her breath or clenching her diaphragm, she can not relax the rest of the body, and will not be able to enjoy the full benefit of these stretches. (See Chapter 3 for more information on the importance of breathing in Thai massage.)

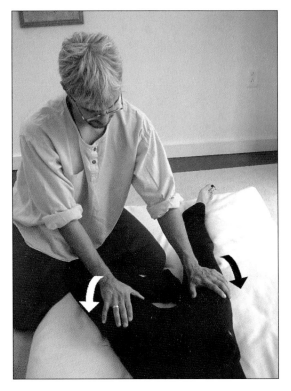

Press with even palm presses on both the client's thighs at the same time. Keep her hips squared and on the mat, and bring her bent knee down towards the floor.

With those who are less flexible, the bent leg may not come all the way to the mat. Remember that it is more important to keep the hips square and on the mat than to get the bent knee down to the floor. Use a cushion or prop (or your own leg) under the bent knee if necessary to keep the hips in correct position.

If you have a very flexible client you can place her foot on top of her thigh in the half-lotus position to give an extra stretch. If you decide to use this position, to protect her knee, keep her foot and the ankle straight and engaged.

ॐ **Correlations with Yoga** ॐ

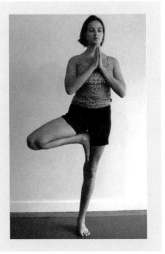

Sanskrit: *Vrksasana*
English: Tree Pose
Points: Engage standing leg with hip over ankle; place bent leg foot as high up on leg as possible; hip bones spread; navel stays forward; take bent leg knee out to side
Benefits: Stretches groin, hips, chest and shoulders; strengthens legs, abdominals, calves, knees, ankles, arches of feet; relieves sciatica; improves balance
Contraindications: Headache, low blood pressure

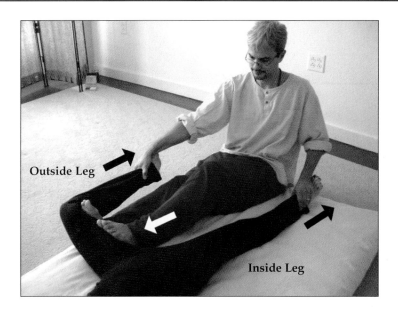

19. "Paddleboat" on Line i3

Take hold of the client's straight leg with your inner hand. Use your outside foot to bring the client's outside leg into a 90° angle. For this step, you may have to adjust your position from that which is shown, depending on how long your legs are and how long your client's legs are. If necessary, you can hold all the way up at the knees. The important thing to remember is keeping her bent leg at a 90° angle with your feet.

With your inside leg, apply a little bit of pressure to her outside leg hamstring by straightening out your knee. Press right along the midline of the back side of the leg. This is probably your first contact with line i3. (See Chapter 3 for more details on this meridian.)

The important thing to keep in mind with this step is body mechanics. Don't use your upper body muscles. Simply anchor yourself by holding the client's legs, and lean back. The foot press is achieved simply by straightening your bent inside leg, as if you were in a paddleboat. Bending and straighten your leg to apply foot presses, walk along the back of her thigh.

If you are comfortable in this position, try walking with both of your feet. Walk along the back of her thigh from the knee as far up as you can toward the groin and then back down. Do this a couple times.

Be sure to apply your feet carefully on the back of her thigh. Think of the foot press like the palm press, where you stretch out you fingers to achieve an even distribution of body weight over a wider area. This isn't a heel press, or a press with the ball of the foot. Nor should you use the outer blade of your foot, which would split the hamstring over the femur. Be sure to flatten your foot out so that sole of your foot is evenly distributed.

If you have a client who may enjoy deeper pressure, you can do a heel press here once you have warmed up the hamstring as explained. After a heel press, you can cool it down with more walking.

When trying to do this step with less flexible clients, as always take care not to hurt them. If they can not bend the hip to a 90° angle, skip this move. There are other ways of accessing line i3 that we will be looking at shortly.

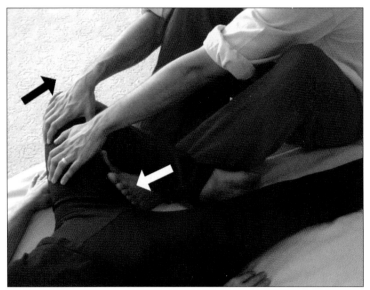

20. Pull on Line o1

Stop walking along i3 in the middle of the thigh. Release the client's straight leg, take hold of the bent leg with both hands, and fold the bent leg across the tops of your feet so that the client's shin is against your shin.

As shown in the photo, your shins keep the client in the figure 4 position while your feet apply pressure into her hamstrings.

Bring your hands around and reach for line o1, hook your fingers in, and lean back. Release, and repeat, following line o1 from the knee to the thigh.

This stretch may not be possible for everyone, so if they can not do it, just skip it. If yourself are not flexible enough to do this step as shown, try with only one of your feet.

21. "Thai Fist" on Lines i1 and i2

Finish this section with the Thai fist, patting along lines i1 and i2 along the inner thigh to relax the muscle before moving on.

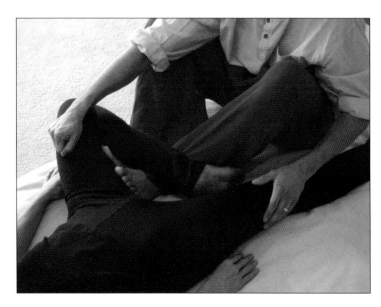

22. Leg Traction

From the same position you have been in for the last two steps, take a hold of the client's leg and bring it up as in the photo, at a 90° angle with the shin parallel to and the thigh perpendicular to the ground. Bend your inner knee, and place your outer leg so that it is straight and flat against the ground. (If you use a bent leg for this step you will be unstable, and if your leg slips while pulling back you could injure your client.) Your foot should support the client's thigh.

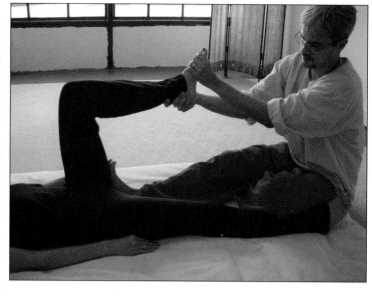

Now, push her knee toward her chest, spread out your toes, and place your your foot evenly down onto her thighs as shown in the first photo. Your entire foot should be flat and fully contacting the back of her thigh.

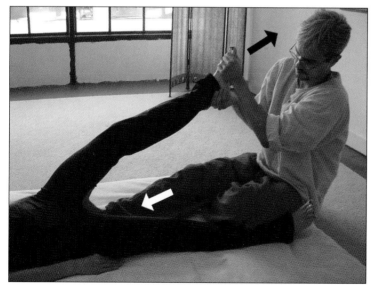

Next, hold the client's foot with two hands, and lean back as shown in the photo to the right. As her leg straightens out, the ball of your foot hooks onto her sit-bone to immobilize the torso, and as her leg is pulled, you give traction to the hip, knee, and ankle.

With your hands positioned as in Step 6, bring the foot twist to the outside, then change your hand position and bring the foot twist to the inside. Repeat two or three times each. Be gentle, and don't be surprised if you get a pop from the hip with some clients.

To release this position, bring the client's leg back to the 90° position in which you started.

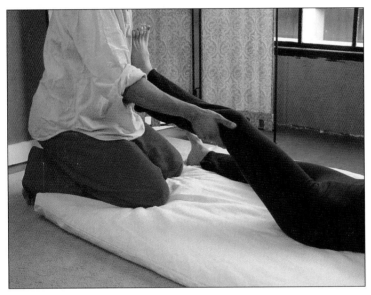

23. Shake Leg to Relax

Shake the client's leg gently to relax the hip. Scoop your hand under the knee, lift up to bend the knee, and then release it quickly. Do this several times as you position yourself for the next step.

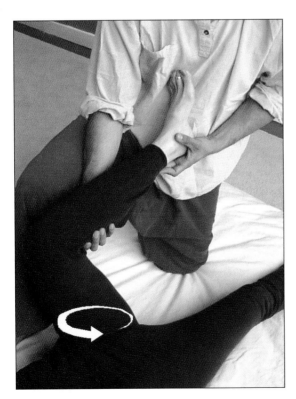

24. Hip Rotation

Bend the client's knee to a 90° angle, with the shin parallel to the ground. Bring yourself in close to the client, bending your outer knee and resting on your inner knee. As always, don't use your upper body strength for this step. With the proper stance here, all you do to rotate the hip is to hold the bent leg at the 90° position, and rotate your own hips. Rotate the client's hip through the entire range of motion, five times clockwise and five times counterclockwise in circles of increasing size.

This is a hard move for many clients, who are hesitant to give up control of their hips. If your client is clenching her muscles when you are trying to do this step, shake the leg gently and encourage her to relax the hip and try it again. Just a little gentle shake is usually all it takes to get a client to relax. Have the client breathe deeply into her abdomen and learn to enjoy giving up control for a little while.

25. Hip Stretch (Flexion)

Bring the client's leg back to the 90° starting point you used for the previous step. This time put your outer palm just outside of her shin, and put your inner palm on the top of her foot. (Remember, you should never apply pressure to the knee itself, and never apply pressure on bone.)

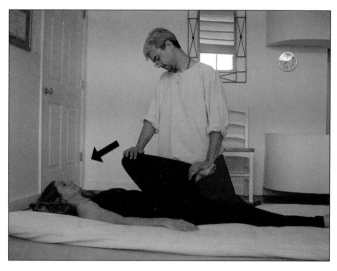

By leaning your body weight forward, keeping your back straight, and moving from your hips, slowly bring her knee towards her sternum. In this position, you want to stretch her shin, all the way down to the ankle and the top of her foot.

This is a great stretch for the iliopsoas, or hip flexor, but as with most steps, it is more important to keep the hips square than to achieve the full stretch shown in the photo. As with any of the steps in this book, if the client can not reach as far as shown, simply take her to where she can go, and encourage her to relax. Beware that I am showing in all photos the ideal for these positions. Every client may not be able to reach this ideal, but you should always keep the picture of the ideal and be working towards it.

You may have to encourage your client to breathe in order to help her relax. If she is holding her breath, this will lock up the abdomen, and this will prevent her hip from stretching as deeply as it could.

If you suspect that there may be some history of knee injury, do not do this step. A modification to protect the knees is to put your forearm in the pocket of her bent knee to provide a little bit of space for the knee to expand as it bends. This is particularly helpful with a less flexible client.

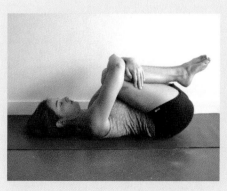

ॐ **Correlations with Yoga** ॐ

Sanskrit: *Pavana Muktasana*
English: Wind-Relieving Pose
Points: Long spine, forehead towards floor; sit–bones towards heels
Benefits: Stretches muscles of lower back and spine; improves digestion & elimination
Contraindications: Pregnancy, abdominal pain, hernia, severe depression

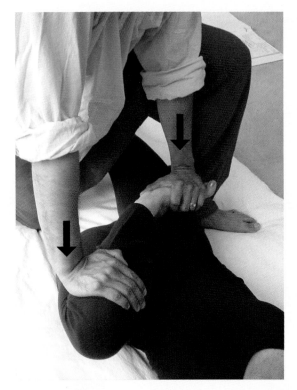

Alternate Method: Pigeon Pose
This posture is slightly different, and you can either use it in addition to or instead of Step 25.

In this move, the knee is brought not towards the sternum, but towards the outside. Care should be taken in positioning the ankle for this move. Be sure that the ankle is straight, and that the stretch is applied evenly across the top of the foot.

Apply your body weight down through both your hands, being careful as in Step 25 not to overstretch the client's knee. (You can insert your forearm into the bent knee in this step as well.) This time, the client should feel this stretch in the hip and groin, rather than in the iliopsoas.

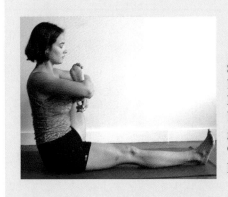

ॐ **Correlations with Yoga** ॐ

Sanskrit: *Eka Pada Rajakapotasana* Preparation
English: One-Legged King Pigeon Preparation
Points: Long spine; foot engaged; straight back
Benefits: Stretches quadriceps, inner thighs, groins, hip flexors, abdomen, chest and neck
Contraindications: Lower back pain, knee pain, ankle pain

26. Hamstring Stretch

Next, straighten your client's leg and again bring her knee towards her chest for a hamstring stretch.

This stretch focuses on the insertion of the hamstring, not on the back of the knee. The idea is not to straighten the client's knee completely (as shown in the yoga pose below), but to bring the knee as close as possible to the sternum, and then to attempt to straighten out the leg.

Remember to use your body weight, and not your upper body strength, to position the client. This is a challenging move for the therapist to perform with correct body mechanics, and there are different options depending on your height and the length of the client's leg. Where you position yourself relative to her leg will come with experience.

Apply your body weight and bend into your forward knee to achieve this stretch. The idea is for your client to relax in this move, so if you see her tensing up, encourage her to keep breathing deeply, which will relax the hamstrings.

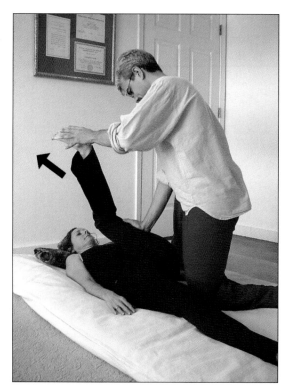

ॐ **Correlations with Yoga** ॐ

Sanskrit: *Supta Padangushtasana* Variation
English: Reclining Hand to Foot Pose Variation
Points: Sacrum remains level to floor; engage quadriceps muscles
Benefits: Stretches hips, quadriceps, hamstrings, groins, calves; strengthens knees; relieves mild backache, sciatica, and menstrual discomfort
Contraindications: High blood pressure (raise upper body on blanket), headache, diarrhea

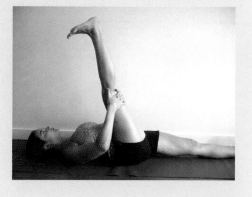

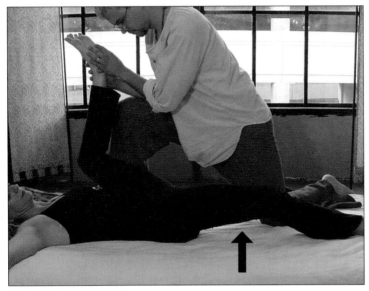

Incorrect Alignment
This photo shows a common mistake when performing Step 26. Therapists must keep an eye on the straight leg as well as the leg that is stretching. The straight leg should not be allowed to rise like the client's is in this photo. This throws off the alignment of the hips.

Correct Alignment
In this photo, the problem is corrected by applying the therapist's hand to the client's upper thigh. Apply weight evenly through both your arms and hands to keep her straight leg flat against the ground while her stretching leg moves towards the sternum. This keeps the pelvis and the hips in correct alignment.

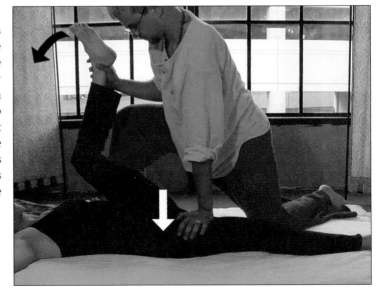

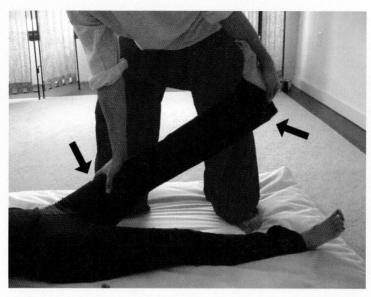

Alternate Methods for the Hamstring Stretch

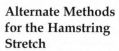

This page shows two alternate ways of performing Step 26. For the less flexible client, the move is changed slightly. The top photo shows the therapist's hand cupping the client's heel and the therapist's forearm placed against her foot. To stabilize her leg, place your other hand on her thigh. As you lean forward, your forearm stretches her foot towards her head, engaging the calf and hamstring. Be careful not to hyperextend her knee in this position by applying too much body weight to her upper thigh.

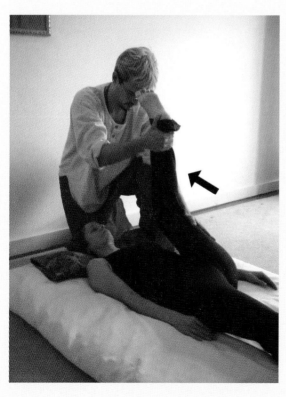

The second photo is an option for your more flexible clients. Squatting or kneeling behind the client's head, hold the heel and pull it towards you. You can support her thigh with your other hand so that she doesn't roll from side to side.

A drawback to this variation is that you are not able to stabilize the non-active leg, so this move should only be performed on those who are flexible enough to stretch this far without raising the straight leg. That little bit of space under the client's straight leg in the photo is the maximum that you should allow.

27. Hip Stretch
(Lateral Rotation)

Now, take the client's bent leg and put it into the pocket that is made by your bent leg. Allow her hip to fall to the outside a little. From this position, apply your body weight down through your straight arms and "cat paw" hands.

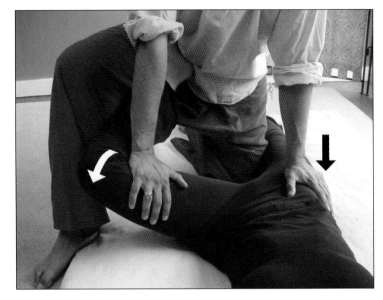

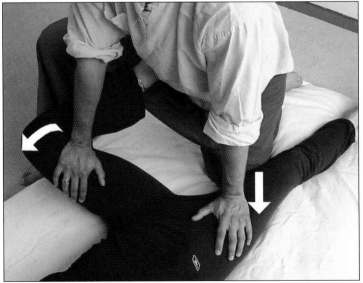

This photo shows another view of the same movement. As in Step 26, your inner hand keeps the client's straight leg flat on the ground to keep her hips square. Your hand on her bent leg applies gentle pressure with palm presses.

Remember, as in all steps, for proper body mechanics your back should always be straight and your hips should always be square. Apply the stretch mostly just by bending into your forward knee.

Again, as with Step 26, be sure not to allow her straight leg to rise from the ground.

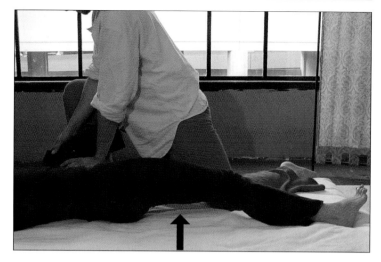

Keeping your inside hand on her straight leg will allow for the correct alignment of her pelvis and hips, and deepen the stretch. Note how much less I can stretch her hip when she is in proper alignment. However, this stretch is much more beneficial than the one shown above.

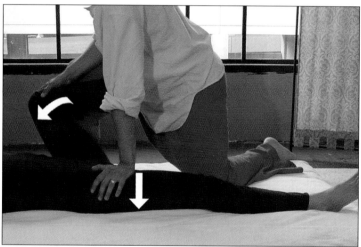

ॐ Correlations with Yoga ॐ

Sanskrit: *Virabhadrasana II* Variation
English: Variation on Warrior II
Points: Knee directly over ankle; tailbone tucked in; sternum lifted
Benefits: Stretches muscles of the ankle; strengthens back, leg, foot and abdominal muscles; relieves mild backache, sciatica, and menstrual discomfort; improves balance; increases stamina; prevents osteoporosis
Contraindications: Heart problems, high blood pressure (modify with hands on hips)

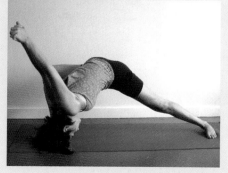

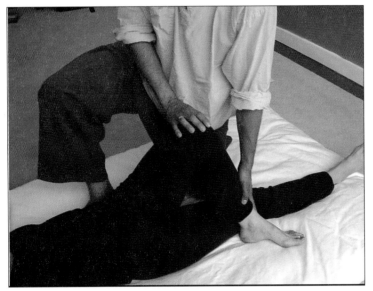

28. Spinal Twist

Now, take the client's foot and place it to the outside of her opposite knee. Next, slowly apply pressure to bring her bent knee down towards the ground. Place your hand or foot in the client's arm pit to create a stretch that crosses the body. (Using your hand is shown below, using your foot on the following page.)

Hold the client in position for five breaths.

The purpose of your foot or hand in the armpit is to keep her shoulders square. The focus of this stretch is the lower back, so you don't want to let the client's shoulders come off the ground. Keeping your hand or foot firmly on her upper body prevents any lift, but be sure to press only on the pectoral muscles so as not to injure your client. If you are applying pressure on the upper arm instead, her upper back may start to lift, causing strain on the front of the deltoid and pectoral muscles.

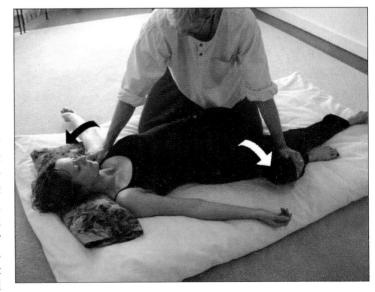

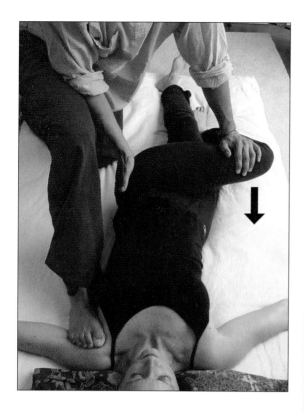

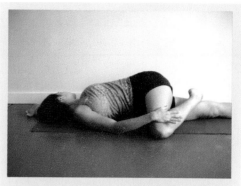

ॐ **Correlations with Yoga** ॐ

Sanskrit: *Shava Udarakarshanasana*
English: Spinal Twist (Lying)
Points: Take knee to floor only if sacrum remains comfortable, taking care not to overstretch; both shoulder blades on floor
Benefits: Stretches and strengthens muscles of spine; stretches sacroiliac joints; relieves mild backache
Contraindications: Severe back pain, spinal injury

If someone is more flexible, once her knee is down to the ground, put a hand on her hips or the small of her lower back and gently pull her over for a little extra twist.

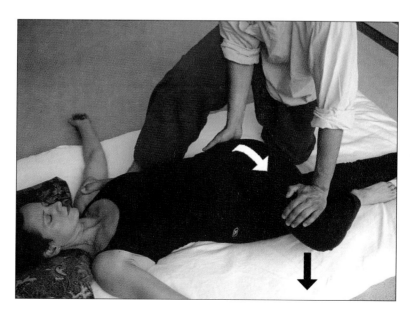

29. Quadriceps Stretch
(Medial Rotation of Hip)

From Step 28, you should be able to take a hold of the client's bent leg ankle and bring the heel back to the glutes as shown in the photo to the right.

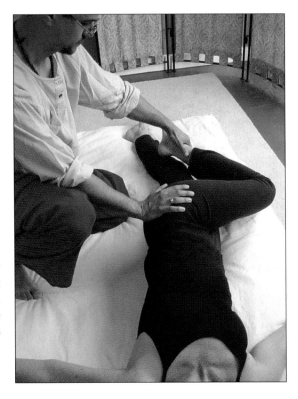

Supporting the leg in one hand and her hips in the other, gently roll her back down so that her back is again on the mat. Be sure that the client's heel remains close against the glutes during this transition, as shown in the photo below.

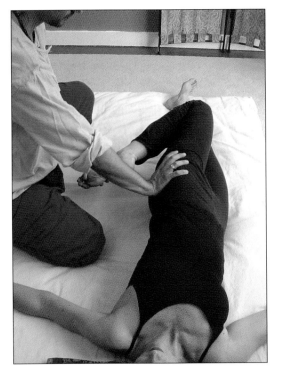

Once the client is in position, apply palm pressure to the bent leg, gently stretching the quadriceps muscle.

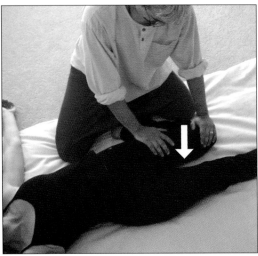

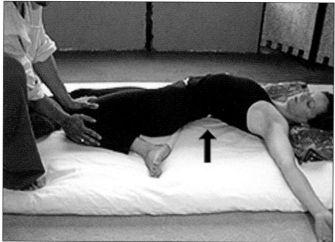

Most clients will not be able to perform the stretch as shown in the yoga pose below. Very few people will be able to rest on the tops of their feet while keeping the hips square, and the back solidly on the ground.

If the foot is not able to tuck under the heel completely, the lower back will arch as you try to bring the bent knee down to the mat, as shown in the top photo. What you want to do in that case is to support the client's knee with your own knee, as shown in the second photo. Rest her knee on your own leg, and focus on keeping her hips on the mat. Concentrate not on lowering her knee, but on squaring the hips.

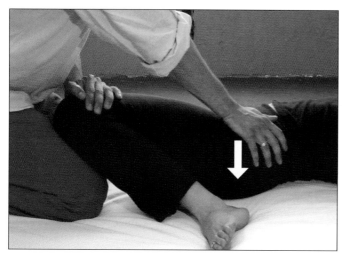

IMPORTANT: It is critical that you release this position by retracing the steps you took to get your client into it. First, roll the client back onto her side. (You can't pull the foot out of where it is without injuring the knee!) As you lift her hip off of the mat, her leg will naturally open. Once her leg has released, support it and bring her back down onto the mat.

ॐ Correlations with Yoga ॐ

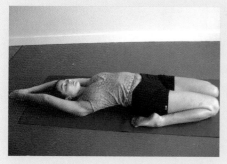

Sanskrit: *Supta Virasana*
English: Reclining Hero's Pose
Points: Bent knee at midline; bent-knee heel brushing side of hip
Benefits: Stretches abdomen, quadriceps, knees, hip flexors, lower back and waist; reduces menstrual discomfort; aids in digestion; relieves asthma;
Contraindications: Knee pain, ankle pain, lower back pain, high blood pressure

Advanced Variation: Finger Press Iliopsoas

This is an optional move you may wish to consider with your clients who enjoy more pressure and deeper work.

In Step 29, the iliopsoas muscle is exposed and engaged. It is easily accessible by using a bladed hand to finger press just inside the pelvic girdle.

Press down gently in synchronization with the client's breathing. As the client breathes in, release the press to allow her to take a full breath. As she exhales, press down deeply into the muscle.

Be sure to press on the iliopsoas muscle, and not on the colon or the hip bone.

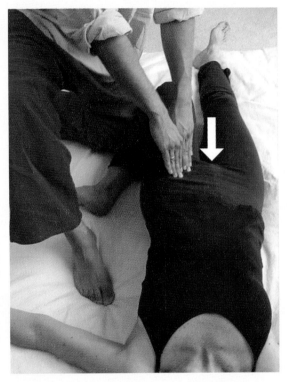

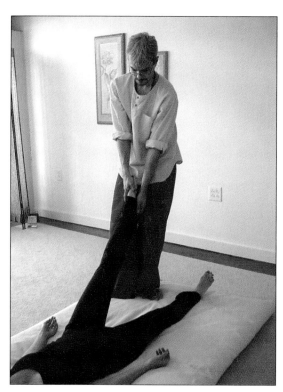

30. Shake Leg to Relax
Take a hold of the client's foot, and give it a good shake to relax all the muscles.

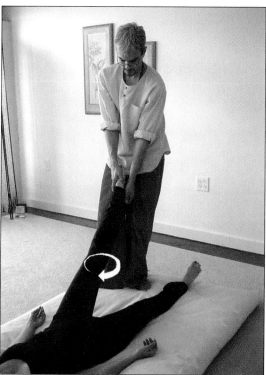

31. Rotate Hip
Now, rotate the hip clockwise and counter-clockwise.

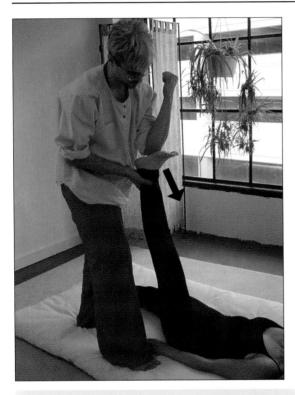

32. Hamstring and Calf Stretch: Elbow Press of the Foot

Bring the client's leg up—ideally to 90°. This next step is a hamstring stretch which targets the back of the knee by keeping the leg totally straight as you apply pressure to the foot.

First, warm up the hamstring by pushing the client's toes down towards the body. Next, press the nine foot points with thumb presses. For more pressure, use the forearm roll, or do an elbow press on those nine points.

With all of these presses, start with the points closest to the heel and work towards the toes, so as to increase the hamstring stretch gradually.

ॐ Correlations with Yoga ॐ

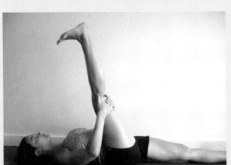

Sanskrit: *Supta Padangushtasana* Variation
English: Reclining Hand to Foot Pose Variation
Points: Sacrum remains level to floor; engage quadriceps muscles
Benefits: Stretches hips, quadriceps, hamstrings, groins, calves; strengthens knees; relieves mild backache, sciatica, and menstrual discomfort
Contraindications: High blood pressure (raise upper body on blanket), headache, diarrhea

33. "The Splits" (Abduction of Hip)

Bring the client's leg back down to the mat. Slowly swing the leg out to the side, gently testing how far it can go. When you reach the maximum point, hold the leg there and plant your feet as shown in the photo to keep both her legs straight.

As in other moves we have seen, If you go too far with this stretch, the client's opposite hip starts to lift off the ground. If this is the case, you can apply pressure to the upper thigh with your inside hand to keep the hips square and the thigh on the ground (such as

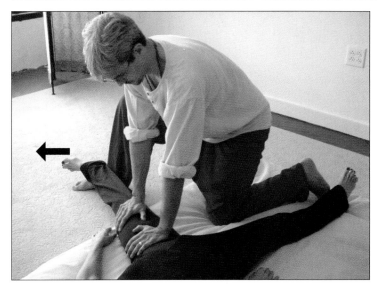

with Steps 26 and 27).

Apply palm presses to the inside of the active thigh on line i2 along the groin muscle. Cover the entire area of the inner thigh, from the knee to the hip and back. Be gentle as you proceed, because as you press directly on the groin muscle you will find that some of these points can be quite sensitive.

Alternate Method for More Flexible Clients

This alternate method for more flexible clients is similar to that for the hamstring stretch (Step 26). Go around to the outside, hook the active ankle with your foot, and apply palm presses along the inner thigh. Again, this step is only for clients whose non-active leg does not begin to rise from the mat.

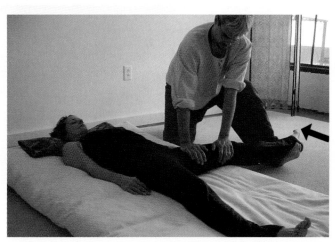

ॐ Correlations with Yoga ॐ

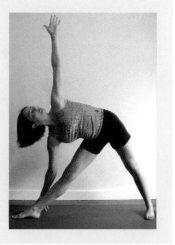

Sanskrit: *Utthita Trikonasana*
English: Extended Triangle Pose
Points: Back toes angle to front of mat 10°; engage both quadriceps; spread hip bones; lengthen both sides of rib cage; head directly over front foot
Benefits: Stretches muscles of the legs, knees, ankles, shoulders, chest, spine; strengthens thighs, knees, ankles; relieves mild backache, sciatica; prevents osteoporosis
Contraindications: Heart trouble, high or low blood pressure, headache, diarrhea, serious back injury, neck problems (don't turn head)

34. Cross Stretch
(Adduction of Hips)

Stand up, walk the client's leg up to 90°, and bring it down on the opposite side.

Plant your inner knee right next to her thigh above her non-active knee to keep that leg in place. Hook her active leg onto your outer ankle again.

The ideal is to take her foot to her outstretched hand. (See photo of yoga pose below.)

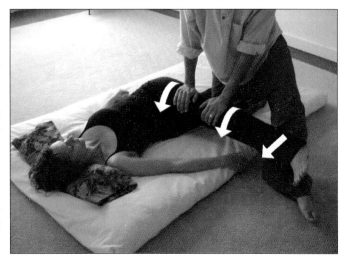

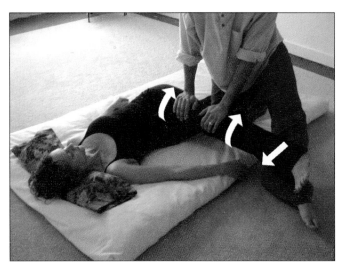

Holding this stretch you can do a palm press of the active leg (shown in top photo). The palm press is in the direction of the stretch, just on the outside of the thigh, covering the thigh from the knee to the hip and back.

For an extra stretch, pull towards you along i1 as shown in the photo to the left. Start from the knee, move all the way up to the hip flexor (iliopsoas), and then work your way back down.

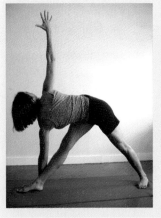

ॐ Correlations with Yoga ॐ

Sanskrit: *Parivrtta Trikonasana*
English: Revolved Triangle Pose
Points: Back toes angle towards front of mat 45°; engage both quadriceps; take front leg hip back to square with back leg hip; level sacrum; lengthen spine; shoulder blades towards spine
Benefits: Stretches muscles of the legs, hips, spine, and chest; relieves mild backache; improves balance
Contraindications: Spinal injury, severe back pain, low blood pressure, headache, diarrhea

35. Shake Leg to Relax
Release the previous stretch, and walk the leg back to 90°. Shake the leg out to relax it and to make sure the pelvis and back are straight and aligned. Set the leg down.

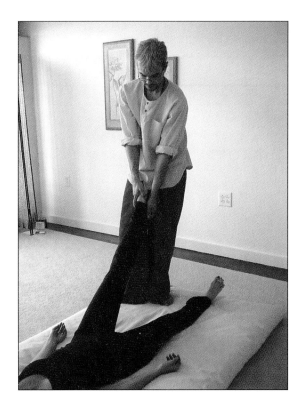

Repeat Steps 17-35 for other leg. Finish leg routine by palm pressing both legs. (See Step 9.)

Hands and Arms

36. Thumb Press Palm Points

Walk around to the client's side. Start with the left hand for a female, or the right hand for a male.

Isolate the client's middle finger using the last two fingers of each of your hands. Place the client's hand flat on the mat. Position yourself in correct posture, placing your body weight over her hand, keeping your arms straight. While simultaneously drawing her hand open by pulling up with your fingertips, apply thumb presses to her palm.

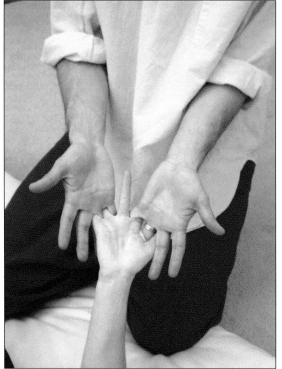

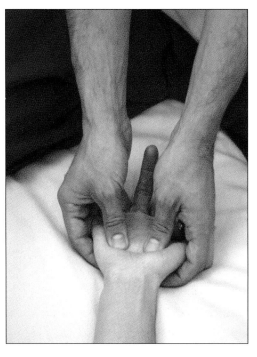

There are nine points on the palm which roughly correlate with the nine points on the sole. Press them one at a time or two at a time. The top level points are right under the knuckles. The middle level points are in the middle of the palm. The bottom points are at the base of the hand.

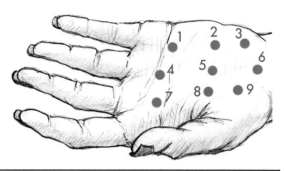

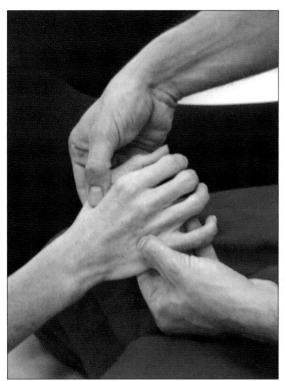

Roll the hand over. Very gently thumb press or thumb circle the two points on the top of the hand. These two points are sensitive acupressure points. The point by the thumb is located between the thumb and forefinger, in the webbing in-between where the bones of the two fingers meet. The second point is just below and in-between the knuckles of the fourth and fifth fingers.

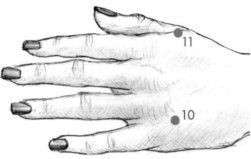

37. Thumb Circle Back of Hand

As you did with the feet, apply gentle thumb circles starting from the top of the wrist in the region of the carpal tunnel. Thumb circle gently, following the tendon of each finger, down to the first knuckle.

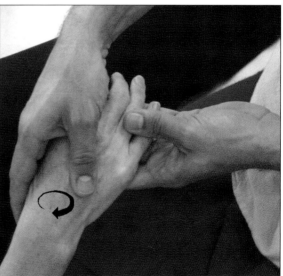

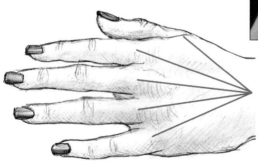

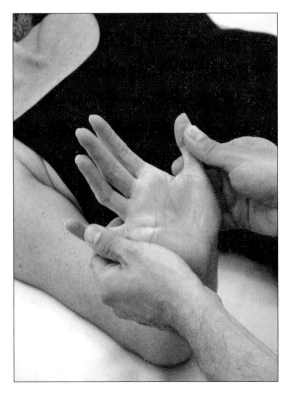

38. Stretch Palm & Fingers

Start at the base of the client's palm. Run your thumbs all the way along the hand and out to the ends of the pinky and the thumb at the same time. Pull back the thumb and pinky together in order to stretch out the whole palm. Start back at the base of the palm, and this time run your thumbs up to the index finger and ring finger at the same time. Lastly, start at the base of the palm and go up the middle of the hand to the tip of the middle finger.

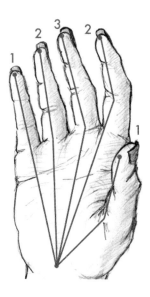

39. Pull Each Finger and Crack Knuckles

Start with thumb circles on each knuckle to warm up it up. Take each individual finger and rotate it around both directions. Apply a little bit of traction to the finger by gently pulling. Move laterally to medially, from the pinky to the thumb.

Make sure that you do not run along the sides of the fingers. Your grip should hold across the top and bottom of the fingers. This way, you can squeeze tightly without hurting.

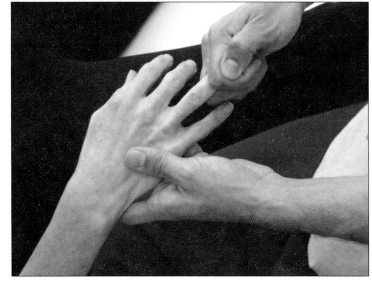

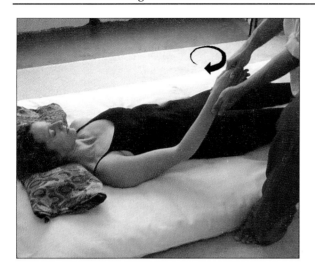

40. Rotate Wrist
Gently rotate the wrist, clockwise and counterclockwise. Hold the wrist with one one of your hands, and the fingers with the other, so as to support the joint while mobilizing it. (This rotation can also be done by interlocking your fingers with the client's.)

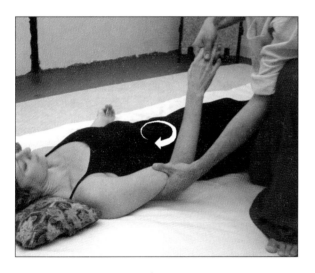

41. Rotate Elbow
Rotate the client's elbow, holding above the elbow on the upper arm to both support and immobilize it.

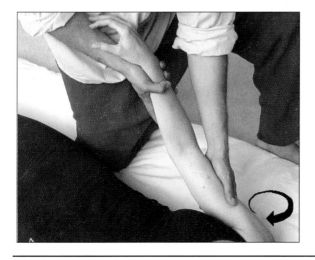

42. Rotate Shoulder and Shake Arm to Relax
Holding the upper arm, rotate the shoulder both clockwise and counterclockwise several times in each direction. Next, shake out the arm to relax it.

43. Stretch, Palm Press, and Thumb Press Outer Arm *Sen* Line

The steps for the arm lines are very similar to those for the legs. We will be performing the same three steps for the arms as we did for the leg meridians in the A-B-C-B-A pattern: stretch, palm presses, and thumb presses.

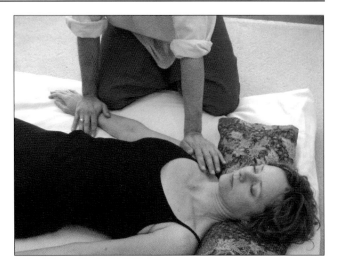

Kneeling beside the client, bring her arm close to her body in order to keep it aligned. To stretch the arm, place one of your palms on the top of her hand and the other palm on the top of her shoulder. Use a butterfly position for your hands and lean forward a little bit while applying even pressure. Next, palm press from her fingers to her shoulder and back. Now, work the o1 meridian with thumb presses, moving from her fingers up to her shoulder and back. Finish by repeating the palm press and stretch.

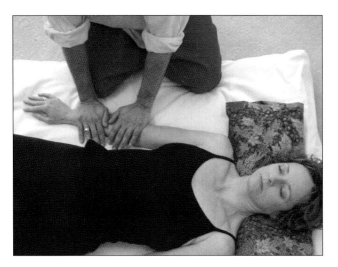

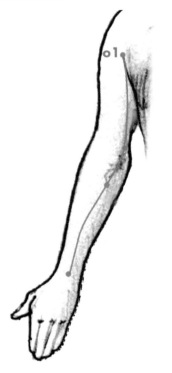

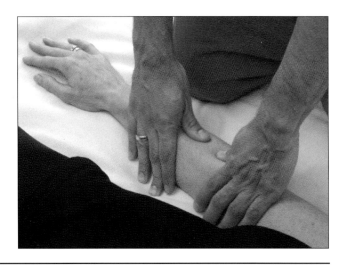

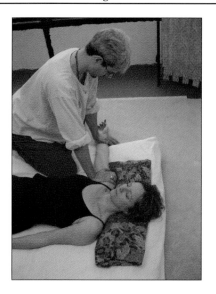

44. Stretch, Palm Press, and Thumb Press Inner Arm *Sen* Lines

Bring the arm out to a 90° angle, and adjust your posture to face the client's arm. Again, start with the stretch. Place one of your hands on the client's palm, and the other hand on her arm pit, and apply a little body weight to align her arm. Next, palm press from fingers to shoulder and back. Then, thumb press the meridians. Move along the outer branches first, moving from wrist to elbow and back. Then go up line i1 up the midline of the forearm, up the upper arm, all the way to the armpit, where you gently press, and then come back down. Finish the A-B-C-B-A pattern by repeating the palm press and stretch.

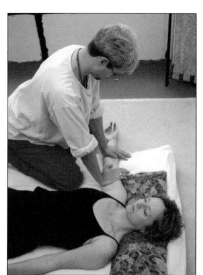

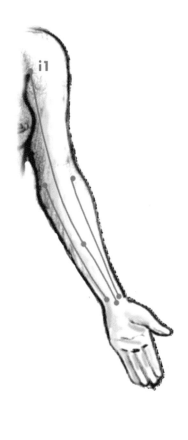

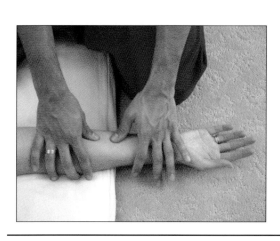

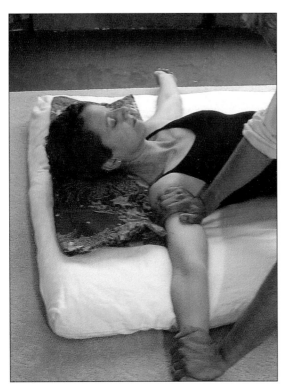

45. Palm Press and Blood Stop

Starting at the client's hand, palm press up to the armpit. Then, place your hand at the brachial plexus, at the point where you feel the brachial pulse. Apply solid, even pressure to this point with your palm while holding the client's arm steady. Hold this blood stop for 10 seconds, and then release. As the blood rushes back down the arm, palm press with both your hands back down to the fingers.

46. Pull Arm to Stretch

Stand up. Pull the client's arm in all directions to stretch out the shoulder and elbow.

Don't pull so hard that the client's back lifts from the mat. If someone is too light, put your hand or foot on her shoulder to keep her back securely on the mat as you stretch her arm.

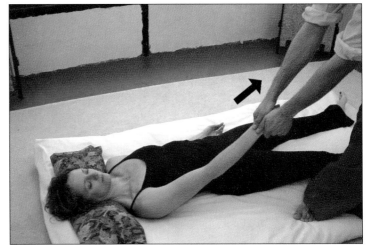

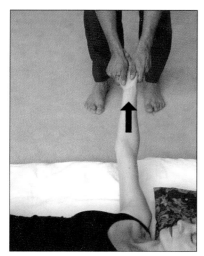
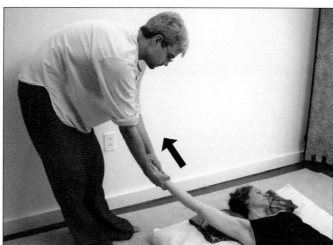

47. Medial Arm Pull

Cross over your client and pull her arm across her chest. Hold one of your hands on her shoulder to keep her scapula on the ground while your other hand grips her hand or wrist. Pull her arm while pressing into her shoulder.

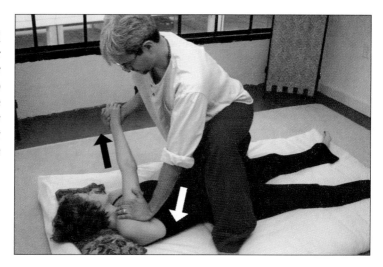

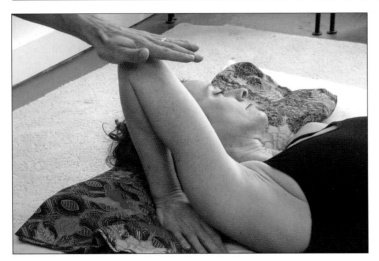

48. Stretch the triceps

Bring the client's arm up into the position shown in the photo. Plant her palm so that her fingers are pointing towards the shoulder. In this position, as you apply the pressure to the elbow, the wrist will straighten out rather than strain.

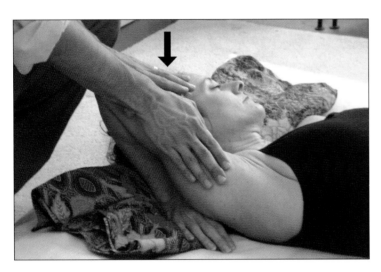

Once the arm is in this position, palm press along the triceps.

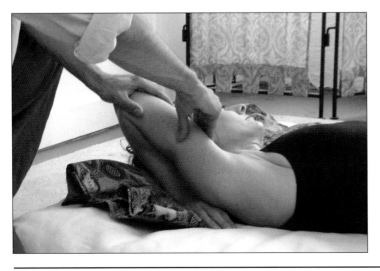

Then, thumb press along o1. Finish by repeating the palm press and stretch before releasing the arm.

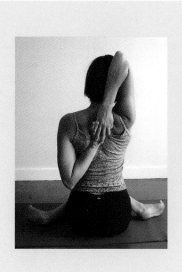

ॐ **Correlations with Yoga** ॐ

Sanskrit: *Gomukhasana*
English: Cow-Face Pose
Points: Both sit-bones grounding, keep top arm rotating so inner arm faces the ear; bottom arm shoulder blade towards spine, spread collarbones and lengthen back and neck
Benefits: Stretches hips, quadriceps, ankles, shoulders, triceps, and chest
Contraindications: Shoulder injury, neck injury, hip injury

Alternate method for less flexible clients

If a client can't bend her wrist as depicted in Step 48, have her cup the back of her neck with her palm, and perform the movements as described. This will not be as deep a stretch as shown in the photos of Step 48, but is just as effective for those that are less flexible.

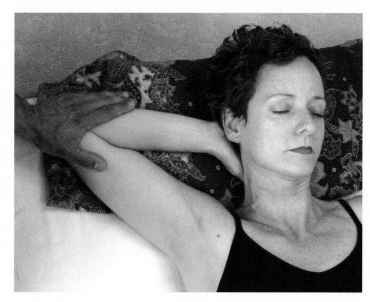

49. Palm Press Arm Above Head

After the intense stretch for the triceps, bring the client's hand and arm straight above her body and palm press from the wrist to the shoulder and back. This will open the shoulder and relax the triceps.

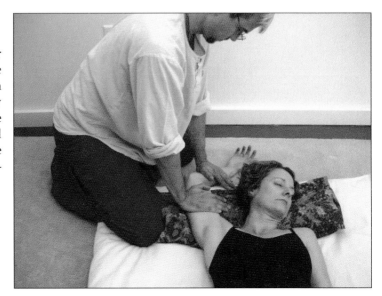

50. Shake Arm to Relax

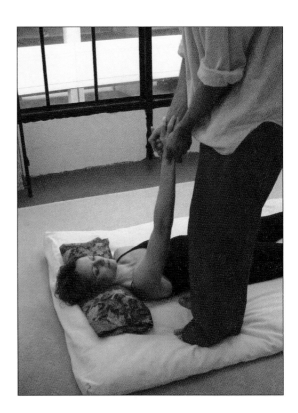

Repeat Steps 36-50 for Opposite Side

The Abdomen

51. Finger Press Under Clavicles

Leave your client's arms at her sides. Make sure to lay her out so her shoulders are even and her arms fall evenly and naturally against her sides with palms facing up (*savasana* pose again). If you feel comfortable doing so, straddle your client in order achieve the best mechanical advantage. Position your body weight over her torso, which is where you will be working.

Use straight fingers, straight wrists, straight arms, and maintain a straight back. Press with your body weight just under the client's clavicles. Your fingertips will fit neatly into the depressions just above the pectoral muscles. These are sensitive acupressure points that stimulate the upper respiratory tract. Start medially at the shoulders and progress towards the sternum. Stop before the sternum, so as not to press on bone, and then move laterally back to the shoulders. Finish by applying pressure to the same area with palm presses.

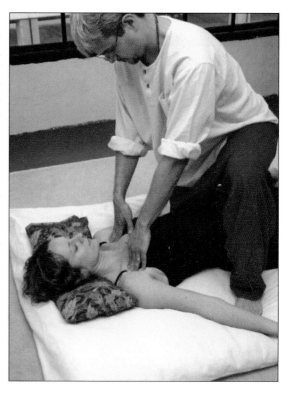

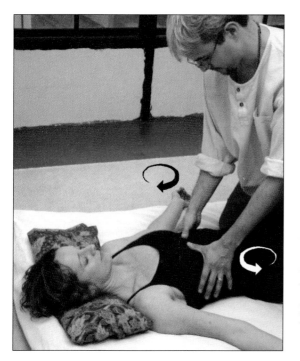

52. Finger Circle Rib Cage

This step provides a general massage of all of the intercostal muscles, the muscles that are holding the ribs together. You can access these muscles with finger circles in between each rib.

Note that massage work on the front of the torso does not follow the bottom to top guideline. Instead, beginning just under the clavicles, move laterally to medially, draining towards the heart. Follow the contour of each rib, progressing downward from the clavicles towards the stomach. Visualize the drainage of energy and lymph towards the sternum or heart.

53. Thumb Press in Intercostal Spaces

Start toward the sternal notch at the base of the neck and move down to the solar plexus. Use a thumb circle to locate the intercostal spaces, and then press lightly with your thumbs.

This step can be a sensitive move on many people, especially women. Be careful not to press on breast tissue.

Finish by applying a little pressure on the solar plexus with your thumb.

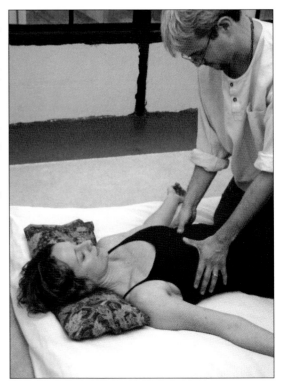

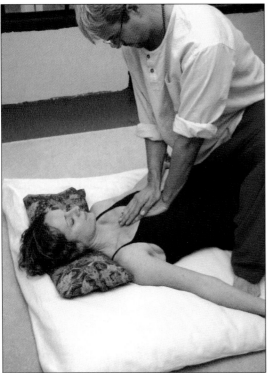

54. Palm Circle and Press on Sternum

Place one palm or two on the sternum. Apply a gentle palm circle. The sternum is actually a joint, so this step encourages flexibility and motion of the joint. Be very gentle, however: this move requires a gentle press downward, not a CPR compression!

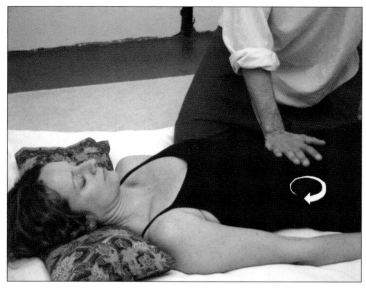

55. Palm Circles on Abdomen

Use gentle palm circles, starting at the client's right hip and moving clockwise in the direction of the colon. You may do one or two cycles around the abdomen, and finish each cycle by placing your hand on her navel and performing a gentle palm press.

The goal of a classic massage should be to use only light contact with the abdomen, which is a sensitive and vulnerable area. The abdomen carries many emotions, and clients can experience emotional releases during this part of the session. Often, the first time I work with a client, I barely touch the abdomen, I just make light contact to establish a relationship and build trust.

56. Thumb Press Stomach Points Around Navel and on Abdominal Muscles

Apply thumb presses to the eight points shown below, one or two at a time. Press gently but firmly into the abdomen. You should feel the client's pulse on either side of the navel. Press and hold these points for 10 seconds each. This is a mild abdominal blood stop, so be sure to avoid this step when contraindicated.

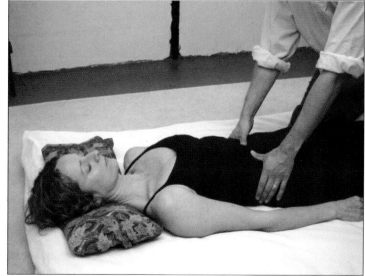

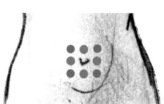

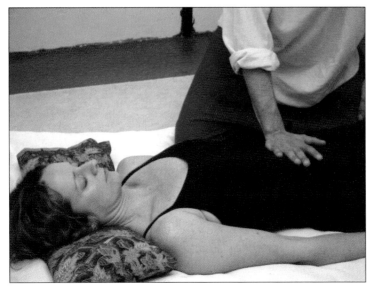

57. Palm Press Abdomen

There are three different techniques you can use on the abdomen, all of which are used in the classic routines in Thailand. However, you may not want to use all three techniques in a single session, at least not unless your client requests that you focus on the abdomen.

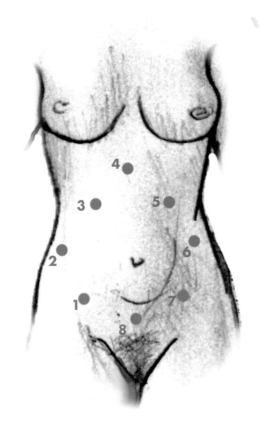

For the first option, follow the eight points shown in the diagram with gentle palm presses. Instruct the client to take a deep breath before each point is pressed. As the client exhales, apply pressure downward into the abdomen. As she inhales, let the pressure off slowly. Move to the next point.

Work your way around the circle, following the course of the colon. You may repeat the cycle a second or third time if your client is comfortable.

In this step, you are following the the colon, assisting in the passage of waste products, and also flushing toxins, lymph, and stagnant energy out of the body.

The second option for abdominal work (at right) is to press on each side of the abdomen with palm presses in two separate circles. Press along the right side first, as shown by the first three arrows in the diagram. Begin at the psoas, proceed up to the solar plexus, and then down underneath the rib cage. Each press should be slow and in synchronization with the client's breathing. Next, perform the mirror image of those same presses on the other side.

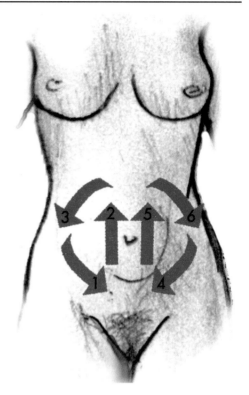

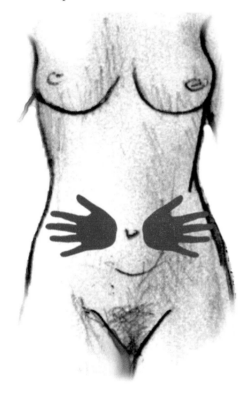

The last of the three options (at left) is to place your palms in butterfly position on either side of the navel. Press first on the right side of the abdomen, then on the left. Each time, palm press slowly in synchronization with the client's breathing. You alternate between each side at least ten times.

Whichever of the three techniques you use, finish by repeating Steps 56 and then 55, to complete the A-B-C-B-A pattern.

ॐ **Correlations with Yoga** ॐ

The variations shown on this page are closely related to the yogic cleanse known as *nauli kriya*. In this exercise, the practitioner alternately contracts the muscles on each side of the abdomen.
Benefits: This practice is considered to be a massage for the internal organs, as well as to improve digestion, excretion, and energy flow throughout the organ systems. It is also considered beneficial for post-partum women.
Contraindications: Heart disease, hypertension, hernia, pregnancy, ulcers

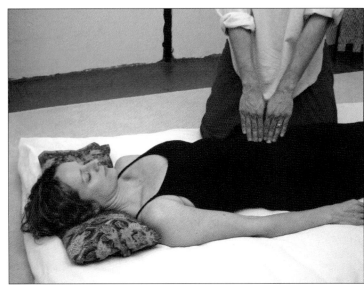

58. Finger Press Psoas

If your client is enjoying the abdominal work thus far, use the tips of your fingers to press along the iliopsoas muscle, just inside the hip bone. Press downward and slightly towards you. Be sure you are working with the muscle and not with the colon, which will be sensitive to this type of pressure.

Finish by finger circling or palm pressing the area to relax it.

If your client feels more comfortable, you may allow her to bend her knees for this step. This takes stress off of the psoas, and allows for deeper pressure.

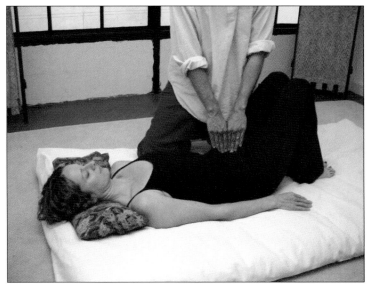

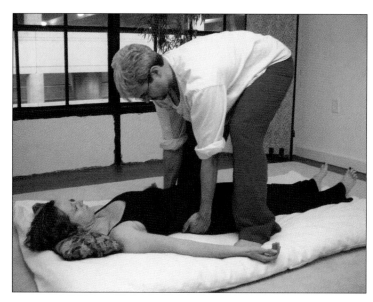

59. Lift From Lower Back
Bring your hands down along the client's sides and work your fingers under the lower back. Gently pull up towards you, preserving the principles of proper body mechanics. This step stimulates the kidneys and the colon from behind.

On lighter clients you can actually lift them up off the ground. Remember to lift with your legs not your back, and be sure to keep the client's head on the ground.

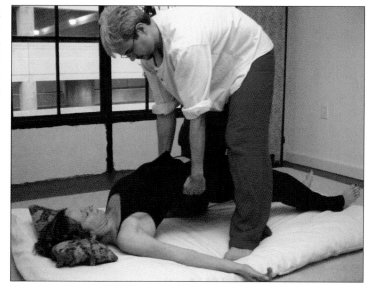

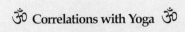

Correlations with Yoga

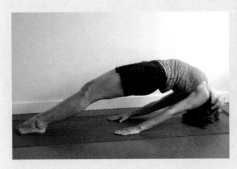

Sanskrit: *Sirshapada Bhumi Sparshasana*
English: Head and Feet to Ground Pose
Benefits: Stretches spine, quadriceps, hip flexors, abdomen, shoulders, neck, and chest; strengthens legs, arms, and wrists
Contraindications: Back or neck injury, weak upper body, high or low blood pressure, headache

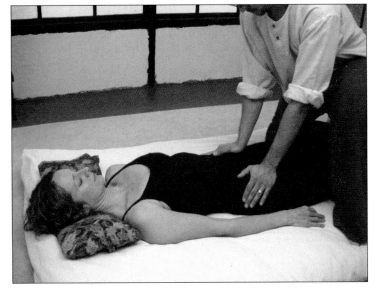

60. Rock Hips to Relax

When you have lowered the client's back down, rock her hips to relax the lower back and iliopsoas muscles. As you rock, try to get some motion in her pelvis and the sacroiliac joint.

Continue the rocking motion down the client's hips and thighs, and finish the abdominal routine by palm pressing down to her feet.

Yoga Stretches

61. Gentle Back Stretch

We have come to the portion of the classical routine which has made Thai bodywork one of the most exciting modalities of massage. Having worked with the meridians and the joint mobilization on the front of the body, we are ready to proceed to the yoga stretches. In this segment of the massage, body mechanics will be a critical concern for the practitioner, and proper alignment will be critical for the client.

We'll begin this segment with a simple back stretch to prepare the back for the work to come. Apply your knees to the soles of your client's feet and your hands to her shins, just under the knees. By bending your knees, move hers towards her head. Don't lift her pelvis from the ground, but do allow her to experience a stretch through the lower back and hips.

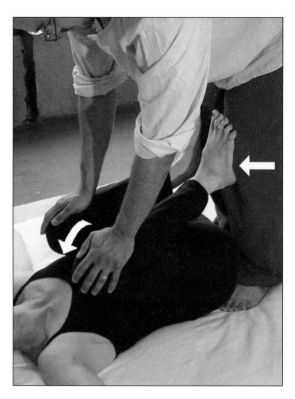

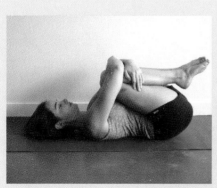

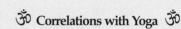
ॐ Correlations with Yoga ॐ

Sanskrit: *Pavana Muktasana*
English: Wind-Relieving Pose
Points: Long spine; forehead towards floor; sit-bones towards heels
Benefits: Stretches muscles of lower back and spine; improves digestion & elimination
Contraindications: Abdominal pain, hernia, severe depression

62. Lower Hamstring Stretch

Making sure the client's back remains aligned and her hips remain square, walk the her leg up to 90° if she can go this far. Bend her right leg (or the left for a male), so that we are working on the appropriate hamstring, and rest her ankle on her opposite knee to keep that leg straight.

Begin to stretch the hamstring by applying elbow presses and/or forearm rolls to the foot. Press along the nine points we used in the foot massage.

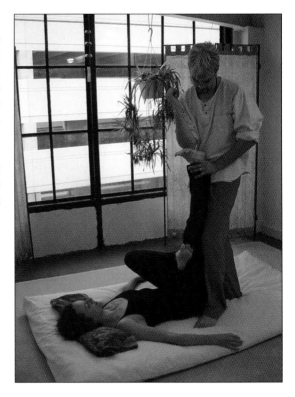

63. Upper Hamstring Stretch

Remove the pillow from behind the client's head.

Next, press her leg forward, pushing her knee towards her chest, and her foot straight over her head. Use your outer hand on her heel and your inner hand at the insertion of the hamstring. With your hands in the correct position, you should be able to perform this stretch strictly with body weight, as opposed to upper body strength.

Advanced Variation for Hamstring Stretch

You may chose to place your leg in front of the client's bent knee to more forcibly straighten her leg. You can use this position for both Steps 62 and 63.

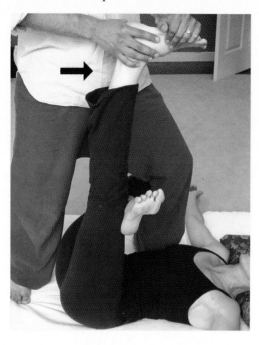

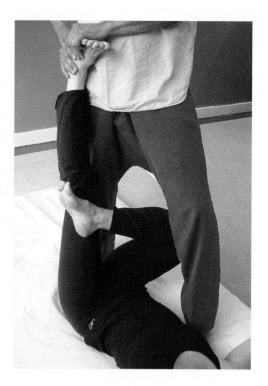

For Step 63, move her leg forward by bending into your leading knee.

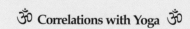
Correlations with Yoga

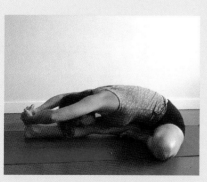

Sanskrit: *Janu Sirsasana*
English: Knee to Head Pose
Points: Foot to inner thigh of opposite leg; ground sit-bones and square navel over long leg; fold forward, revolve same-side ribs away from leg and opposite side ribs towards leg; lengthen spine
Benefits: Stretches hamstrings, groins, calves, spine; strengthens abdomen, spine; improves digestion; reduces menstrual discomfort; alleviates anxiety, stress, and depression by calming nervous system
Contraindications: Knee pain, asthma, diarrhea

64. Pigeon Pose

From the same position you used for the last two steps, adjust your hands so that your inner hand is pressing on the foot of her bent leg, and your outer hand is pressing on the thigh of her bent leg. Place her straight leg up against your shoulder. Using your body weight, lean forward to apply pressure to stretch both the hamstrings of her straight leg and the hip and groin of her bent leg.

Repeat 62-64 for the other leg

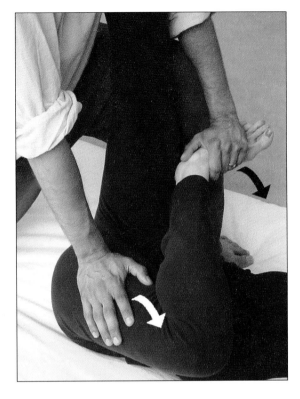

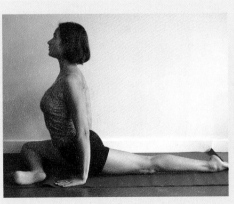

ॐ Correlations with Yoga ॐ

Sanskrit: *Eka Pada Rajakapotasana*
English: One-Legged Pigeon
Points: Long spine; open chest; shoulders back; both hips on mat
Benefits: Stretches quadriceps, inner thighs, groins, hip flexors, abdomen, chest and neck
Contraindications: Lower back pain, knee pain, ankle pain

65. The Plow

Before beginning, make sure the client is aligned properly. Her legs should be together and her back straight. If the client's hamstrings are tight, she will have a tendency to bend her knees as you bring her feet towards her head. To help avoid this urge, have her put her hands on her thighs just above her kneecaps.

Perform this stretch standing at her side, providing support if necessary. First, move her feet towards her head about 45°, bending into your forward leg so as to use the best body mechanics. When her sacrum begins to rise off the ground, slide a hand under to support her and keep her steady. Keep one hand on her sacrum while you bring her legs to the floor behind her

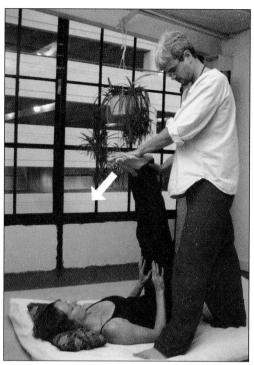

head. Not all clients will reach the floor, and if they do not, you must support their legs so as not to put strain on the back muscles or the spine.

If the client's feet do touch the floor, tuck her toes in, and press her heels away from her head, while maintaining a hand on her sacrum, pulling her back into a straighter line.

Continue to support your client in this pose and have her breathe deeply for five breaths. You must not let the client's head roll to either side, or permit her to fidget in this yoga posture. The neck is extremely vulnerable in this position.

When you feel the client has stretched enough, straighten the her out by retracing the steps you took to come into the pose.

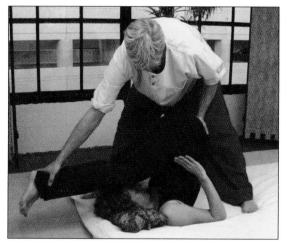

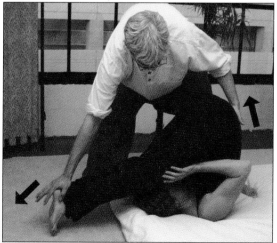

ॐ Correlations with Yoga ॐ

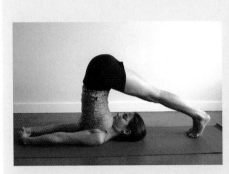

Sanskrit: *Halasana*
English: Plow Pose
Points: Back of head to floor; spine long; collarbones spreading; shoulder blades towards spine; hips over shoulders
Benefits: Stretches hamstrings, calves, spine, shoulders, chest, neck; strengthens muscles of the back; alleviates mild back pain, headache, sinusitis, insomnia; alleviates anxiety, stress and depression by calming nervous system
Contraindications: Pregnancy, neck or shoulder injury, asthma, high blood pressure, diarrhea

Variation for Plow Pose
If your client has very tight hamstrings or back muscles, you may not be able to get very far with the regular plow. In this case, the client is permitted to bend her knees in order to receive some of the benefits of the posture.

Your client will need every bit of support in this posture that she did in the full plow, so be sure to be immediately next to her, and to help her in and out of the posture as described in Step 65.

Over time, clients who uses this pose may wish to experiment with straightening out

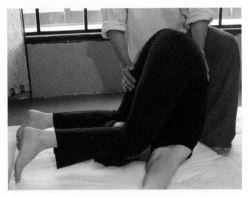

first one leg and then the other. Eventually, they will be able to begin to straighten both legs simultaneously for increasing periods of time.

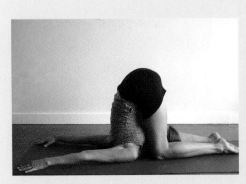

ॐ Correlations with Yoga ॐ

Sanskrit: *Karna Pidasana*
English: Ear Pressure Pose
Points: Back of head to floor, knees towards ears; round spine
Benefits: Stretches muscles of the back and neck
Contraindications: Neck or spinal injury, high blood pressure, asthma, severe depression

66. Butterfly

Before beginning this pose, straighten out the client's back again and make sure her hips are aligned. Hold her legs open at about a 30° angle. Instruct her to spread her arms out to the side, at a 90° angle to her body.

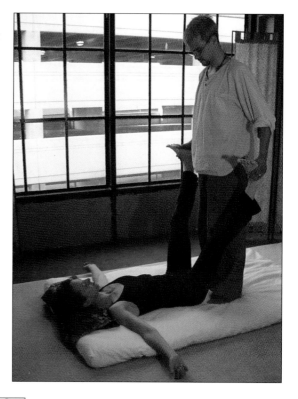

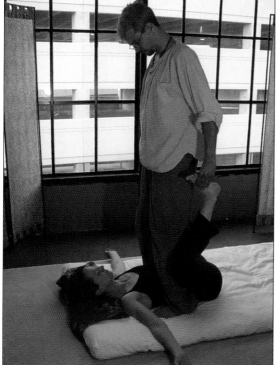

Have her bend her knees a little. Carefully step over her legs, and place each of your feet so it is directly under one of her armpits.

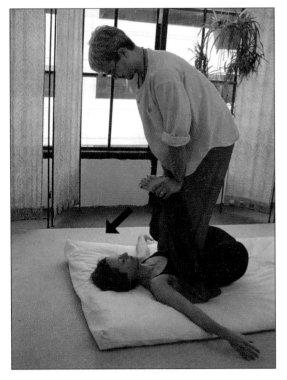

Bring her feet around to the front of your thighs, and hook her heels around your quadriceps. Now, apply body weight to bring her feet closer to her forehead. Bend your knees as the client continues into a deeper stretch. This is not the Bound Angle Pose in Step 70, where the feet go to the navel. In this pose, you are aiming to bring the feet to the ground behind the client's head.

Be sure not to push down into the ground, which would put pressure on her lower back. Rather, push her feet out, towards her head.

Once you have her feet as far down as they will go, hold them in place, and straighten out your legs. This will send her sacrum back towards the floor, and deepen her stretch.

Hold the pose over five deep breaths.

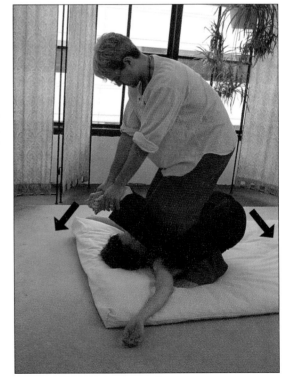

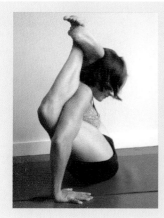

ॐ **Correlations with Yoga** ॐ

Sanskrit: *Dwi Pada Sirsasana*
English: Two Legs Behind the Head Pose
Points: This is an advanced pose and is not recommended without the guidance of a teacher
Benefits: Stretches hips and groins
Contraindications: High or low blood pressure, heart trouble, knee or hip injury

Variation for Less Flexible Clients

This move is especially effective when a smaller individual works on a larger client. Place your feet outside and in line with the client's hips. Kneel on the back of her hamstrings. Keep your knees on the belly of the muscle and tilt them slightly inward so as to keep your body weight steady. Apply your body weight forward, while bringing her feet towards the ground behind her head.

With someone who is larger and less flexible, you are probably going to be able to apply your entire body weight and use the client's muscular tension to keep your balance. If someone is flexible enough that you are in danger of falling forward, you should use Step 66 instead.

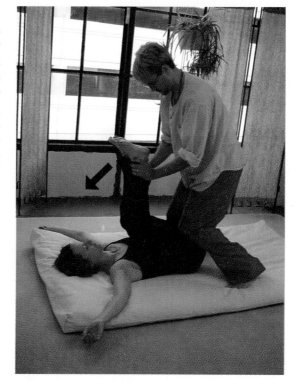

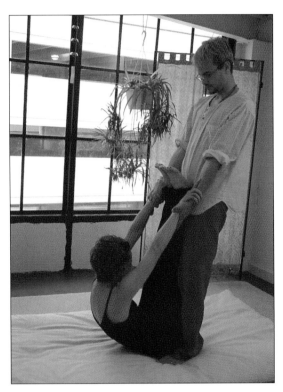

67. Double Leg Pull-Up

Ask the client for her arms and hold each other's wrists. (If either of you have sweaty hands, use talcum powder for safety.)

Be sure to hold your arms in such a way that your palms are facing outward, and her palms are facing towards you. This is the best grip for proper alignment of the client's shoulders.

Gently pull your client up with your body weight, stretching her hamstrings and back. Set her down on the mat, and repeat the pull-up three times, in synchronization with the her exhalations.

(Note this move is not ideal for a heavy client, and you may want to skip ahead to the next step.)

Correlations with Yoga

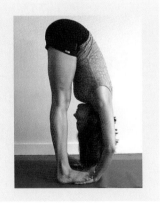

Sanskrit: *Pada Hastasana*
English: Hand to Foot Pose
Points: Engage quadriceps; lengthen spine
Benefits: Stretches backs of legs, upper back; strengthens knee joints, front of legs, and shoulders; relieves headache, mild depression, and anxiety
Contraindications: High blood pressure, heart trouble

68. Cross-Legged Pull-Up

Use your hands to move the client's legs into a cross-legged position as if she was sitting. Ask her for her hands again and use the same grip as for the last step. Do three more pull-ups in synchronization with her exhalation, trying to use your body weight instead of muscle to lift.

On the third pull-up hold the client in position, and start to step your feet backwards.

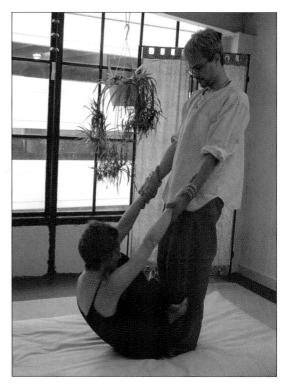

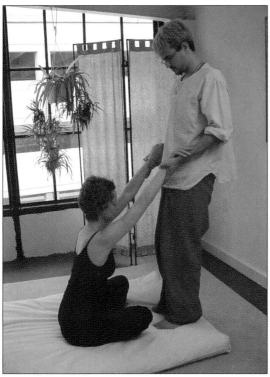

Continue holding hers wrists as you walk backwards, pulling her into a seated position. Finish by setting her palms on the floor.

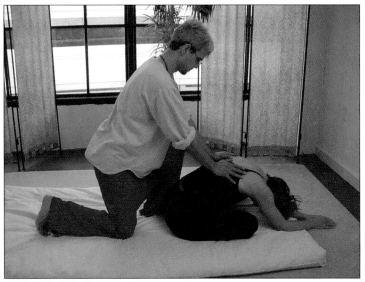

69. Forward Bend with Crossed Legs

This is the first in a series of forward bends. Perform palm presses with "butterfly hands" on both sides of the client's spine, being careful not to press on the actual vertebrae. Starting just above the iliac crest, apply palm presses with your body weight. Your own position should be above the client, so that your back and arms can remain straight.

Continue with palm presses until you reach her shoulder blades. Do not go higher than the shoulder blades, because this will begin to strain the neck.

The object with this stretch is not to bring the client's head to the floor, but to bring her navel to the floor while keeping a natural lumbar curve in her spine.

Stay in tune with your client's breathing, and move with this rhythm.

If your client prefers stronger pressure, use elbow presses or forearm rolls on the back muscles, being sure to never press on bone.

To help her up, put your hand in the middle of her back to keep it straight and put your other hand on her shoulder for support.

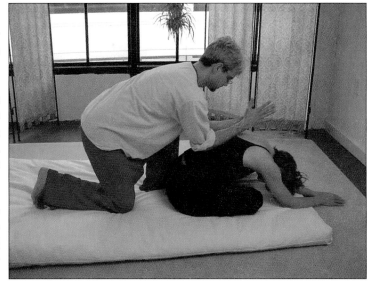

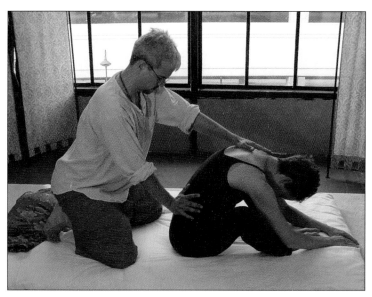

70. Bound Angle Pose

The next in our series of forward bends is similar to the last except for the positioning of the client's legs. Ask the client to put the soles of her feet together, with her heels close to her groin. You may assist here, if necessary.

Use gentle palm presses to bring her back down into a forward bend. Start at the iliac crest and move up to the scapula, then back down. Use palm presses, forearm rolls and/or gentle elbow presses.

To deepen the stretch, ask her to bring her feet in closer to her pelvis.

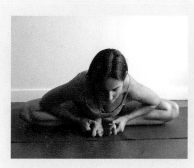

Correlations with Yoga

Sanskrit: *Baddha Konasana* Variation
English: Bound Angle Pose Variation
Points: Skin of inner thigh moves towards knees
Benefits: Stretches groins, hips, and knee joints; relieves menstrual discomfort and sciatica
Contraindications: Knee injury, lower back injury

71. Forward Bend with Straight Legs

Straighten out the client's legs. Bring her feet together, encouraging her to keep her knees straight and toes pointed up.

Apply palm presses, forearm rolls, or elbow presses as you did with the other forward bends.

In this pose, be vigilant that the client does not bend her knees, point her toes, or flop her legs out to the side. It is also very important for the client's back and neck to stay straight.

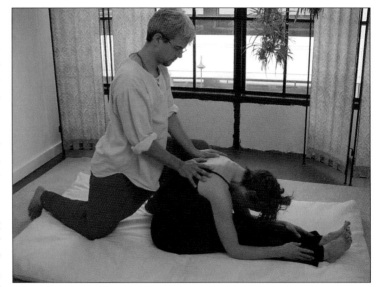

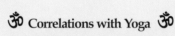

ॐ Correlations with Yoga ॐ

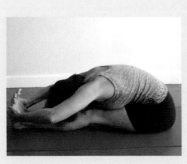

Sanskrit: *Paschimottanasana*
English: Stretch of the West Pose
Points: Engage quadriceps muscles; tilt pubic bone forward and sit-bones backward as you lengthen sternum towards shins, keeping spine long
Benefits: Stretches muscles of the posterior leg and back; strengthens abdomen; alleviates anxiety, stress, menstrual discomfort
Contraindications: heart problems

72. Forward Bend with Wide-Angle Legs

Move to the front of the client and bring her legs out into a wide angle. Ask the client to keep her legs straight and to point her toes towards the ceiling. Remind her to bend from the waist, not the upper back, and to bring her navel to the floor.

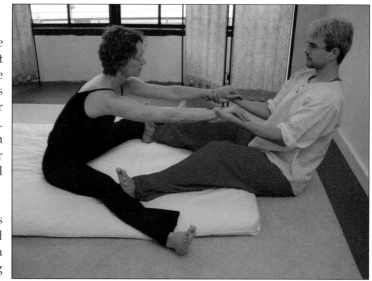

Place your feet on her legs above her knees, and hold each other's wrists. Apply a bit of body weight to bring her into a forward bend. You do not need to press into her legs with your feet, or to pull her arms sharply towards you. Simply applying a bit of body weight in an even, controlled manner will give the client a wonderful stretch.

Hold the client at her maximum over the course of five deep breaths, and then release.

ॐ Correlations with Yoga ॐ

Sanskrit: *Upavistha Konasana*
English: Wide Angle Pose
Points: Engage quadriceps muscles; tilt pubic bone forward and sit-bones backward as you lengthen sternum towards floor, keeping spine long
Benefits: Stretches groins, inner thighs, posterior legs; strengthens spine
Contraindications: Lower back injury

73. Walking Back Stretch

This will be the first of our back-bending stretches. Alignment of the shoulders is critical in all back stretches, and you will have to be sure to keep an eye on your clients during these moves.

Taking the client's arms behind hers back, hold on to each other's wrists. Place your feet under her scapula, and keep your knees bent at 90°. From this position, you should be able to keep your balance using your client as an anchor for your body weight.

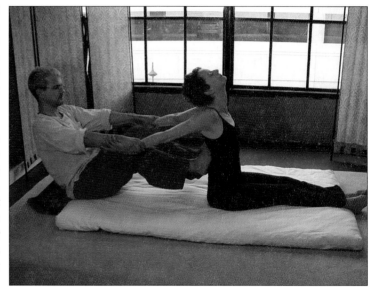

Apply a bit of pressure with the balls your feet, and pull back a bit on her arms with body weight. Press slowly one time, in synchronization with the client's exhalation. Be sure not to dig in your toes, or to press directly on bone. Encourage your client to point her chin towards the ceiling with this step to stretch the neck as well.

Release the stretch, move your feet about 2 inches lower on the client's back, and repeat.

Finish by repeating this stretch one last time with your feet in their original position.

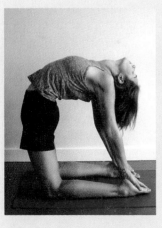

ॐ Correlations with Yoga ॐ

Sanskrit: *Ustrasana*
English: Camel Pose
Points: Inner thighs move towards one another as you tuck tailbone; take shoulders towards ears then down back and towards spine to open chest; round upper back as you slowly descend; release neck if comfortable
Benefits: Stretches spine, quadriceps, hip flexors, abdomen, shoulders, neck and chest; strengthens spine
Contraindications: Back or neck injury, high or low blood pressure, headache

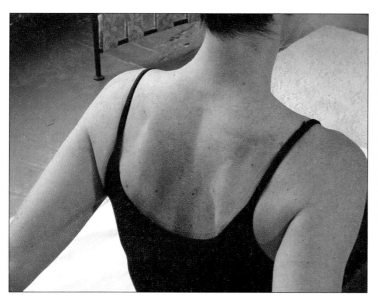

Shoulders - Wrong

Step 73 is the first of several back bends where it is critical to have the client's shoulders in the correct position before moving into the stretch. If the shoulders are rolled forward, as shown in this picture, when you pull straight back on the arms you will compromise the neck and shoulders.

Shoulders - Right

To achieve proper alignment for back stretches, you must rotate the shoulders outward, opening the chest, and bringing the scapula together. (To help my students remember which direction to rotate the arms, I often refer to this move as "revving the motorcycle.")

It is very important to perform this rotation on all clients. However, as you rotate the shoulders, someone with hyperextendable elbows may rotate unnaturally far, potentially causing strain or injury in the posture.

Attention to proper alignment is of utmost importance, and you will have to make the decisions that are best for your client.

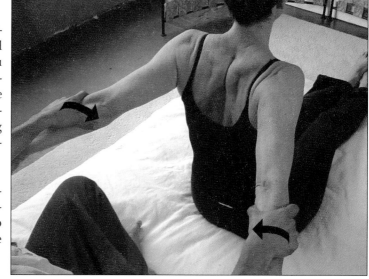

74. Fish Pose

The next pose flows naturally from the walking back stretch. Place your feet against the client's pelvis, and straighten your legs out so that the backs of your knees are completely in contact with the mat.

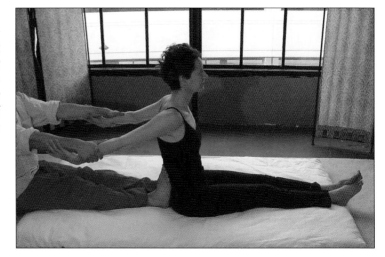

Release the client's arms. Placing your hand on either scapula, help her to lower herself onto your legs.

Place one of your hands on one of her scapulas and your other hand at the base of the client's neck to give her support, while you help her to lower herself onto her legs.

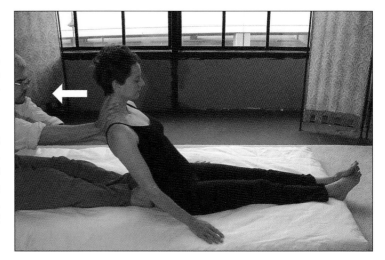

Your toes should provide lift for the lower back. Hook your fingers into the base of the skull, and pull gently toward you to provide traction to the entire neck and back.

Allow your client to relax fully over five deep breaths.

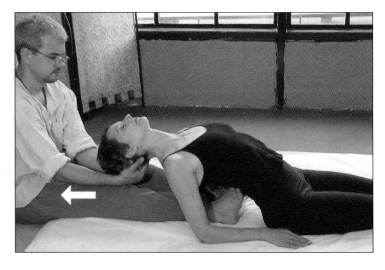

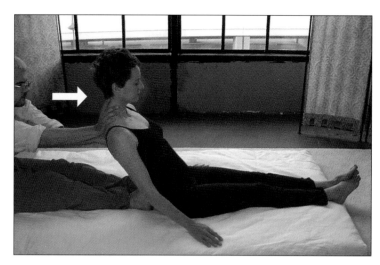

To release this position, retrace your steps, being sure to support her shoulders and neck as you lift the client back up again.

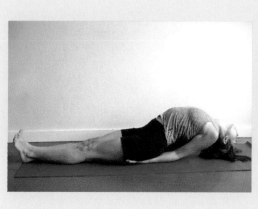

 Correlations with Yoga

Sanskrit: *Matsyasana*
English: Fish Pose
Points: Lift sternum; release neck
Benefits: Stretches hip flexors, abdomen, intracostal muscles, spine and neck; strengthens spine and neck; stimulates digestion
Contraindications: High or low blood pressure, neck or back injury, headache, insomnia

75. Spinal Twist

Instruct the client to cross her legs. The idea for this step is to provide a gentle twist of the back while simultaneously lifting the torso to lengthen the spine.

Place the client's hands behind her head and have her interlock her fingers. The traditional hand-grip is to come through the armpits and hook on to the forearms. If you can not do this on a client, just get under the upper arms at the armpits.

The position of both the client's and the therapist's legs is also important. The photo shows one of my knees on the ground and the other is on the client's leg in order to brace her.

Lift with your arms to straighten her back and open her chest. From this position, rotate the client's torso towards your planted knee to provide a spinal twist. Your knee

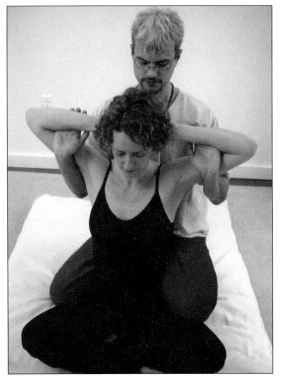

on her thigh will keep the client's leg and sit-bone on the ground.

Come back to center, and repeat this movement three times in synchronization with the client's exhalation. Each time you twist, you can go a little bit further, but be sure her spine stays perfectly erect throughout this step.

Next, switch your knee to the other side, and repeat the movements in the opposite correction.

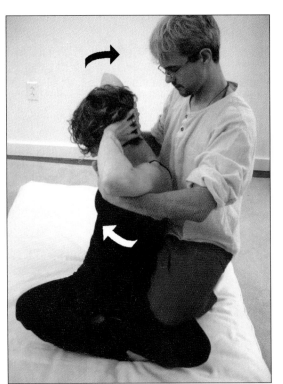

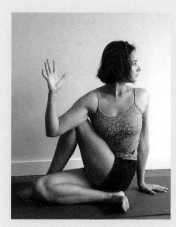

ॐ Correlations with Yoga ॐ

Sanskrit: *Ardha Matsyendrasana*
English: Half Lord-of-the-Fishes Pose
Points: Sole of top leg foot and top leg sit-bone both reaching for floor; back of head in line with sacrum; inhale to lengthen spine and exhale to deepen twist
Benefits: Stretches the shoulders, hips, spine, and neck; alleviates menstrual discomfort, asthma, backache, and sciatica; stimulates digestion
Contraindications: spinal injury, neck injury, diarrhea

Alternate Position for Increased Leverage
You may prefer to perform this movement from a standing position. Use one of your feet to hold down her leg and sit-bone. Lift under her armpits and rotate, holding your straight leg against her back to keep it erect. This allows a better mechanical advantage, especially when working on someone bigger than yourself.

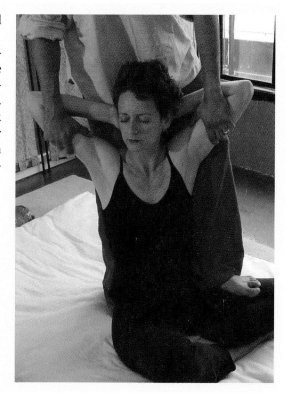

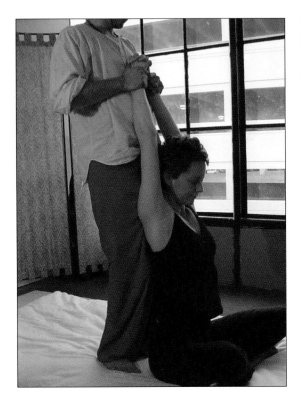

76. Back Lift

Straighten out the client's back by lifting her arms above her head and interlocking her fingers. Hold her forearms. Place your knees just under or on her scapula. Simultaneously lift her arms up, and bend your knees into her back to provide a bit of an arch to the back as it stretches. This step straightens out the spine and relieves any tension from the intense back stretching.

77. Thai Chop on Back

To further relax the back muscles, use the Thai chop along either side of the spine. Start at the lower back, and work upwards to the trapezius muscles. Be sure not to chop too strongly, particularly on sensitive points such as the kidneys. Although it will make a loud noise, the Thai chop should be relaxing and soothing, not at all jarring.

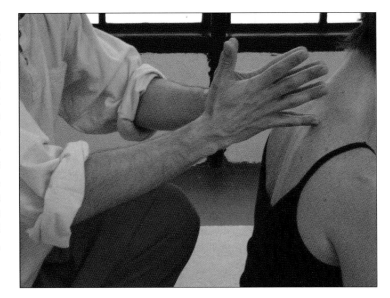

Back

78. Palm Press Feet

Instruct your client to turn over onto her abdomen. I have my clients put the pillow under their chest so that their head can rest comfortably on the mat while their neck remains straight. You may need more than one pillow to make your client comfortable. Also, let her know that she can turn her head to either side.

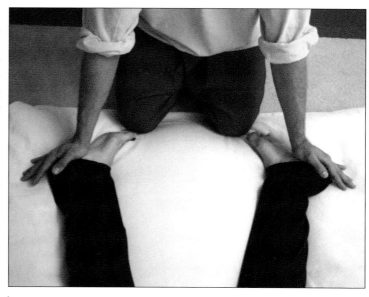

We will start on the back of the body, beginning again with the feet, and working our way up towards the head.

Keep the client's legs just wide enough to kneel between them. Begin with a palm press of the feet.This is a walking palm press from the toes to the heels and back like we did in Step 2. Walk up and down the feet several times.

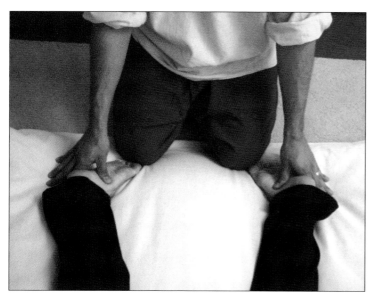

79. Thumb Press Foot Points

Repeat the nine points and the five lines on the soles and arches you learned in Steps 3 and 4. (See diagram on next page.)

Sometimes, a client's arches may cramp up when you press on the feet from this position. If this happens, relieve the pressure by putting her feet on your knees.

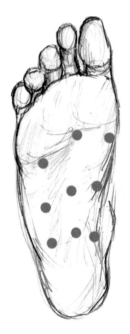
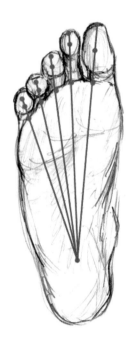

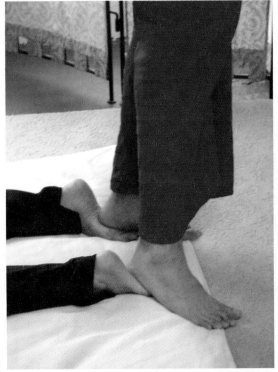

Alternate Method: Foot and Heel Press

For the client who enjoys stronger pressure, use your feet for Steps 78 and 79. Use the flat part of your foot for the "palm press" and your heel for pressing the points. Obviously, the heel is not as precise of an instrument for pressing as the thumb, and you probably will not be able to accurately cover the points and lines depicted above. However, press along the whole sole and arch of each foot and you will be sure to cover all of the points and lines.

This is one area of the body where, for most clients, you can press with the heels without causing pain, but, of course, use caution the first time you perform this variation with a client.

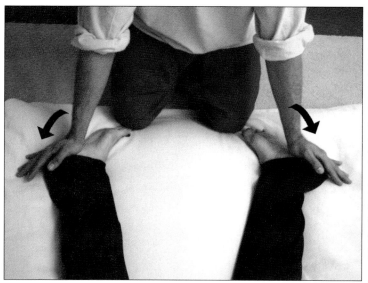

80. Stretch Legs

Stretch both of the client's heels to the outside simultaneously, applying your body weight evenly. Keep your hands in the butterfly position, put them down on the client's heels and lean forward, pushing both of the heels down to the ground.

Make sure the toes are pointed in towards each other and that you stretch the heels to the outside. Do not press the heels in towards the midline.

This is the beginning of the A-B-C-B-A pattern for leg line i3.

81. Palm Press Legs

Palm press the legs, starting at the feet and moving up. This time you can go right through the back of the knee because there are no bones to avoid. Come all the way up to the top of the legs at the insertions of the hamstrings, and go back down. Remember: cat paws, wide fingers, straight arms, bringing your body up over the client, and gently rolling to the outside as you walk up.

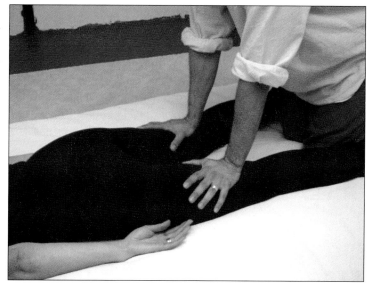

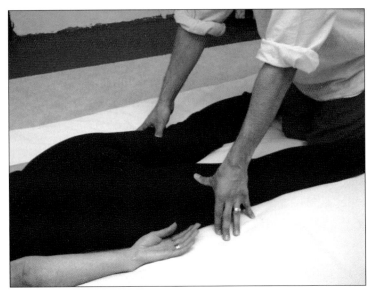

82. Thumb Press Along *Sen* i3

For this leg line, you can work either with both of the client's legs simultaneously as shown, or else with one leg at a time. The meridian goes straight up through the back of the calf, up through the middle of the back of the knee, and up the midline of the thigh. (See Chapter 3 for more detail.) Begin at the Achilles tendon, proceed up to the hamstring insertion, and return once again.

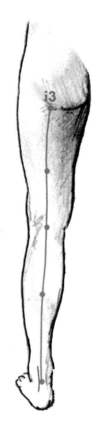

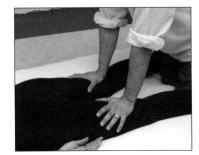

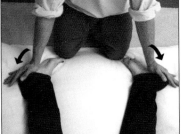

Finish the A-B-C-B-A Pattern by Repeating Palm Press (Step 81) and Stretch (Step 80)

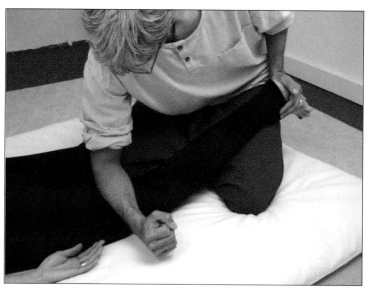

83. Forearm Roll on Upper Thigh

Begin with the left leg for a woman or the right leg for a man. Place the client's shin against your thigh to alleviate any pressure on the client's knee as you proceed with this step.

Apply your body weight down through a 90° arm with a forearm roll. Start behind the knee and work towards the hamstring insertions, go up over the glutes, and up the lower back as far as you can reach while maintaining good body mechanics. Then, work your way back down to the knee. Repeat several times with increasing intensity.

84. Elbow Press Along i3

Use an elbow press on the hamstrings along line i3 for clients who are not too sensitive. Elbow pressing is done by leaning down into your elbow with your body weight. Release by unbending your elbow.

When you are finished with the elbow press, repeat the forearm roll in Step 83 to soothe the muscles.

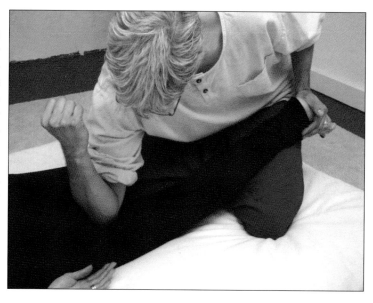

Repeat Steps 83 and 84 for the Other Side

85. Rotate Ankle

Beginning with the left side for a female or right for a male, rotate the ankle from this position. Rotate it five times clockwise and five times counterclockwise.

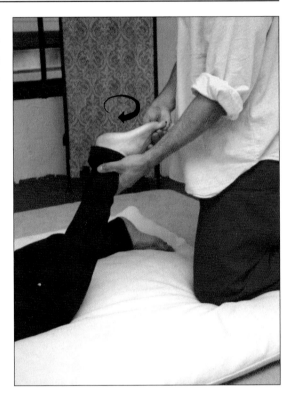

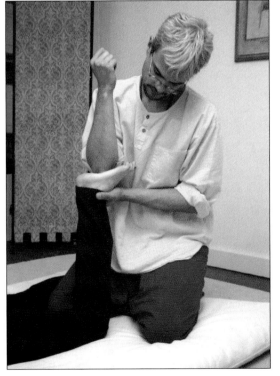

86. Calf Stretch

Bend the knee to a 90° angle. Begin with a forearm roll on the foot to stretch the calf muscles. Next, apply elbow presses to the nine foot points to provide a deeper stretch. Finish by repeating the forearm roll.

87. Knee Flexion

Use your body weight to stretch the front of the client's shin and quadriceps. Place one of your hands on the soft part of the outer portion of her shin, the other hand on the top of her foot. Press her heel into her buttocks.

Stretch the client's leg three times in synchronization with the client's breathing.

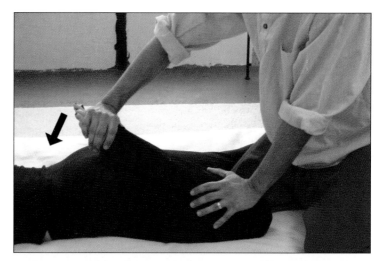

Next, take your hand which was pressing her shin and scoop it under her knee. While again pressing her heel into her buttocks, lift the client's leg off the ground to stretch the quadriceps and hip flexor. Repeat this three times with the client's exhalations.

Repeat Steps 85-87 for the other side.

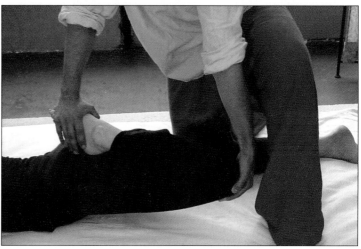

ॐ **Correlations with Yoga** ॐ

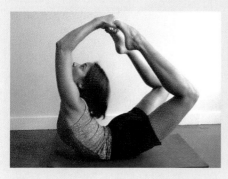

Sanskrit: *Dhanurasana*
English: Bow Pose
Points: Pull on ankles is very gentle to protect knees; inner thighs towards one another; tuck tailbone; spread collarbones and lift sternum
Benefits: Stretches spine, quadriceps, hip flexors, abdomen, shoulders, neck, and chest; strengthens legs, arms
Contraindications: Pregnancy, back or neck injury, high or low blood pressure, headache

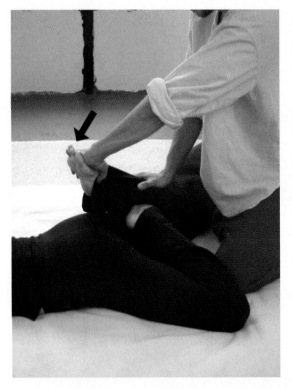

Alternate Methods
There are other ways of performing Step 87, and you can experiment to see what works for you.

The first variation is similar to Step 87, but with the client's ankle behind her knee. This is particularly good if you are concerned about the client's knees and want to provide them with a less intense stretch. Place one of the client's feet behind her opposite knee. Use one of your hands to press her heel toward her glutes, and the other to palm press on the outside of her shin.

The second variation, a double knee flexion, stretches both knees, which gives a lower back stretch as well. This step is for your more advanced clients. Take the client's feet and cross one over the other on the sacrum. Apply your body weight evenly down on the tops of both her feet. Then switch her feet and repeat.

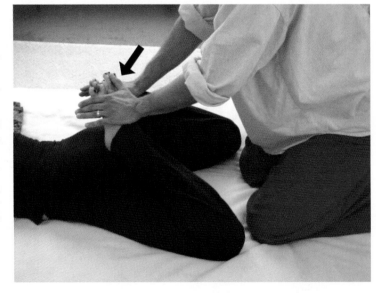

88. Thumb Press Hip Points

Thumb press with a little body weight, or if the client is more sensitive, use thumb circles.

The hip points are shown in the diagram below. There are three points around the head of the femur and three points below the iliac crest.

Press the femur points first, then the iliac points. Always move from the out-side towards the midline of the body. Press right along, but never directly on, the bone.

For this step, you may work with each side individually, or both simultaneously as shown.

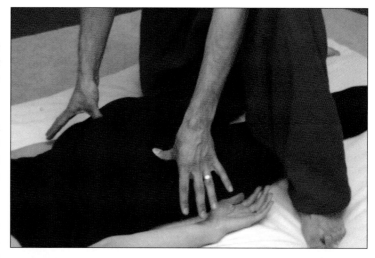

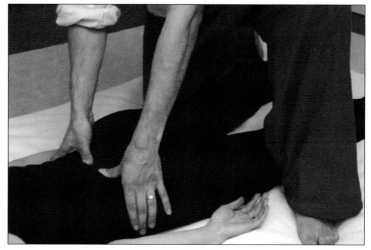

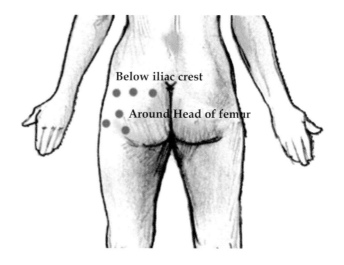

Below iliac crest

Around Head of femur

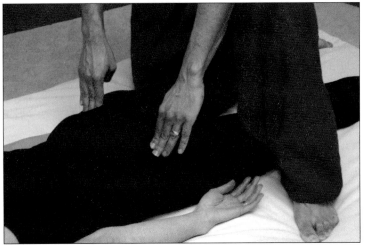

89. Finger Press or Elbow Press Glutes

For this step you will be straddling your client or standing over her for maximum body mechanics advantage. Make sure you press on the soft part of the glutes, away from any bone. Start with finger presses to test your client's sensitivity.

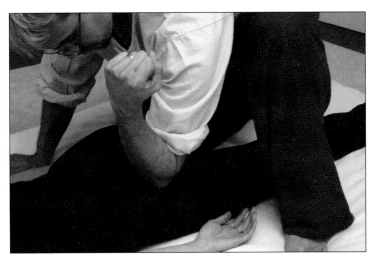

If the client wants more pressure, use the elbow press as well. Lean your body weight in to apply pressure and release by unfolding your arm. When you are finished pressing, cool off the area with a forearm roll.

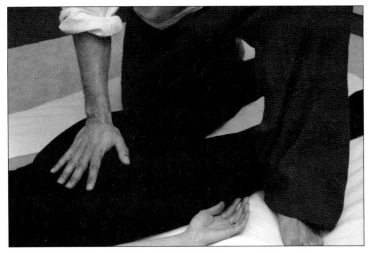

90. Palm Circle Sacrum

This palm circle is similar to what we did with the sternum. Like the sternum, the sacrum is made up of fused bones. Palm circle all around the sacrum.

Don't apply too much body weight as you are pressing on a bone, and always keep a circular motion. Palm, finger, or thumb circles also work well on this type of joint.

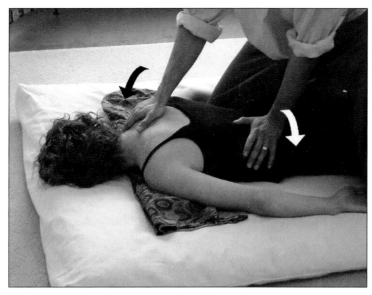

91. Stretch Back

This is the opening step for the A-B-C-B-A pattern on the back meridians. Make sure your client's arms are resting down at her sides, palms up, and that her neck is straight.

This stretch is a nice gentle cross stretch. Place one of your hands up by the scapula, and the other hand in her lower back on the opposite side. Apply a press with body weight, making sure not to press on any bones.

Switch your hands and repeat for the other side.

92. Palm Press Back

As in the forward bends, in this step you will press the client's back with a walking palm press, from the iliac crest to the scapula and back again. Keep your hands in butterfly position, and keep about 2 inches of space between your palms so you are sure not to press directly on the client's spine.

The pressure you use is dependent on the client. Be sure to finish at the scapula, well below the C7 vertebra so that you don't start compressing the neck.

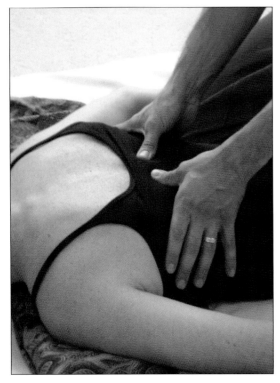

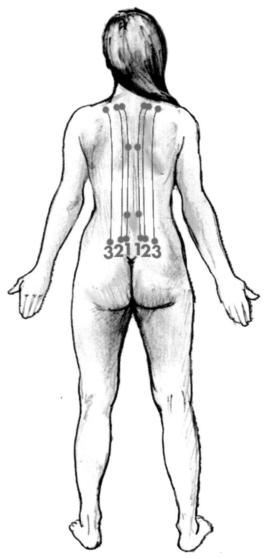

93. Thumb Press *Sen* Meridians of the Back
Following the guidelines in Chapter 3, press the three back meridians with walking thumb presses. Press both **lines 1** together, then both **lines 2**, then both **lines 3**, working from the iliac crest to the trapezius and back again.

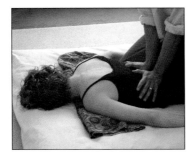

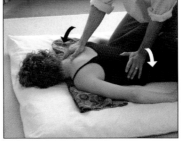

Finish A-B-C-B-A Pattern by Repeating Palm Press and Stretch

94. Palm Circle Rib Cage

Palm circle the rib cage as you did on the front of the body. Again, with the rib cage we ignore the general rule of moving bottom to top. Instead, we start up by the shoulders, and proceed down the rib cage drawing towards the center. Visualize that you are moving stagnant energy and lymph towards the heart. Spread out your fingers and get into the intercostal spaces in between each rib. Circle all along the scapula, the shoulders and the upper arms. Do not forget the latissimus dorsi muscles (the "lats") and under the client's armpits.

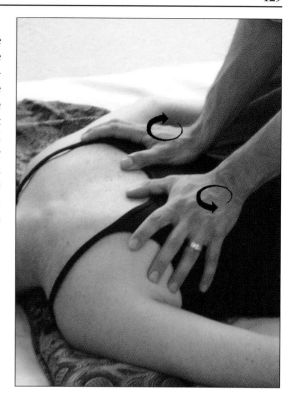

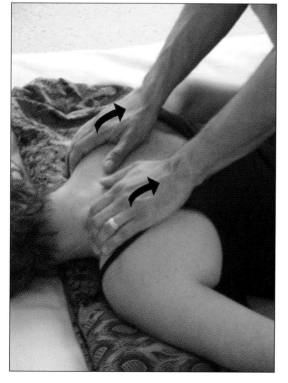

95. Pull Trapezius Muscles

Pull on the trapezius muscles by hooking in your fingers, and leaning back with your body weight.

Start laterally out at the deltoids, and move in to the base of the client's neck.

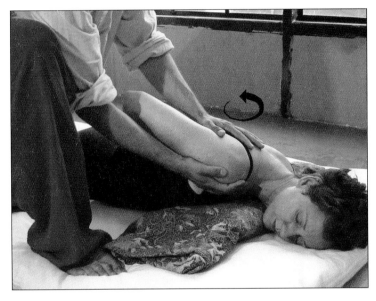

96. Shoulder Mobilization
Start with the left arm for a female or the right arm for a male. Ask the client to turn her head to the same side. Bend the client's elbow, and place her hand behind her back. With her arm in this position, rotate her shoulder first towards you and then away from you. Rotate the shoulder five times in each direction.

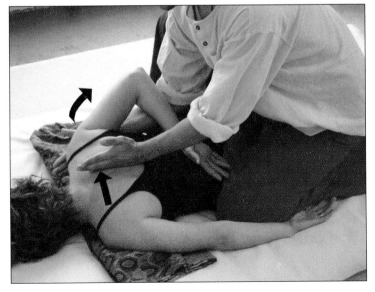

Next, place a bladed hand behind the scapula, and draw the client's shoulder up and towards you while pressing under the scapula. This should be done in such a way that you are stretching the deltoids and the pectoral muscles. The motion here is similar to the opening of the chest and shoulders with the back bends. (See Step 73.)

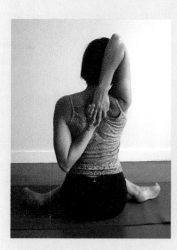

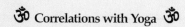 **Correlations with Yoga** ॐ

Sanskrit: *Gomukhasana*
English: Cow-Face Pose
Points: Both sit-bones grounding, keep top arm rotating so inner arm faces the ear; bottom arm shoulder blade towards spine; spread collarbones and lengthen back and neck
Benefits: Stretches hips, quadriceps, ankles, shoulders, triceps, and chest
Contraindications: Shoulder injury, neck injury, hip injury

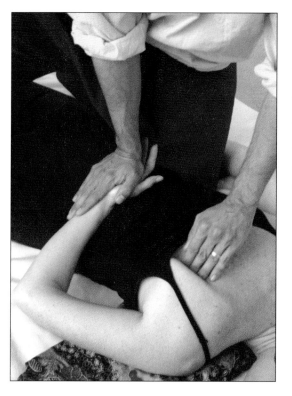

97. Press Under Scapula

Holding the client's hand against her lower back in order to keep the scapula open, finger press or thumb press into the rhomboids underneath the bone. Massage these muscles for a few minutes. They are often one of the tightest areas of the body, particularly with clients who work at desk jobs or other occupations where they are seated all day.

Alternate Method

For clients who enjoy a fair amount of pressure, and whose back muscles are particularly tight, elbow presses on the trapezius and rhomboid muscles are a great option.

Apply pressure evenly and steadily through your elbow, and release by unbending your arm. Apply pressure to the points shown in the diagram below, beginning with the points lower on the body and moving up towards the neck.

You will want to begin and end this move with palm, thumb, or finger circles to be sure to warm up and cool down the muscles.

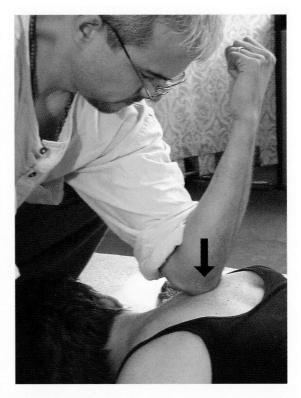

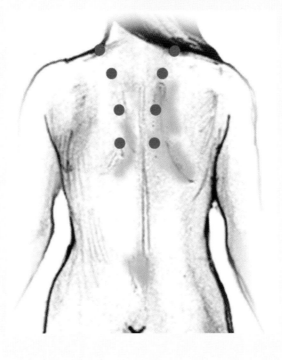

98. Cobra

Bring the client's legs together. Kneel on the client's buttocks so that your knees are in line with her lower back, just above the iliac crest. Allow your weight to rest primarily on her buttocks. Take her arms (at the wrists or at the elbows) and rotate her shoulders to open the chest, as we have done for all back bends.

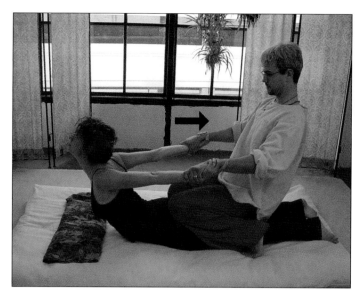

Alignment is very important with this step. If your knees are properly placed, they will prevent the client's back from arching too much and stressing the lumbar spine. (See next page for more details.)

This stretch is performed by gently leaning back with body weight. Do not attempt to pull the client with upper body strength.

When you have reached the proper position, ask your client to point her chin towards the ceiling. Hold this posture over five deep breaths.

ॐ Correlations with Yoga ॐ

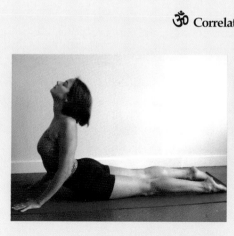

Sanskrit: *Bhujangasana*
English: Cobra Pose
Points: Engage legs; press top of little toes into mat; tuck tail; press evenly into hands; lift sternum; roll shoulder blades back and down spine; lengthen neck
Benefits: Stretches chest, shoulders, abdomen, and spine; strengthens spine and buttocks; alleviates asthma and sciatica
Contraindications: Back, neck, or wrist injury, pregnancy, headache

The cobra is one of the most famous steps from the classical routine. Unfortunately, it is also most often taught incorrectly.

With the cobra stretch, as with all back bends, it is of utmost importance to understand the proper principles of alignment. These include the necessity to rotate the client's shoulders into correct position by "revving the motorcycle" (as shown in the photo in Step 73).

These also include the proper stabilization of the client's pelvis to avoid injury to her lower back. All too often, the cobra is performed both in Thai massage and in yoga classes in such a way that undue stress is placed on the lumbar spine. Performing the cobra as shown in the photo at right, or kneeling way down on the client's hamstrings, will leave her lumbar vulnerable to injury.

As a Thai massage therapist, you must be aware that the cobra is in fact a stretch for the thoracic spine, shoulders, and chest as opposed to the lower back. In order to immobilize the lumbar region and isolate the upper back, kneel directly on the buttocks of your client.

Although your weight will be placed directly over her pelvis, your knees should be above the iliac crest, preventing the lumbar region from lifting off the mat. As you pull back, notice how the client will stretch from the thoracic region in a nice even curve.

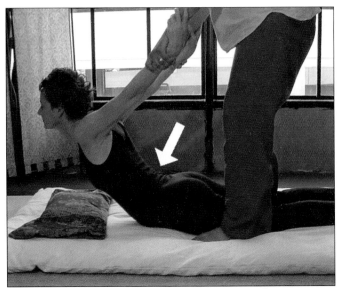

Cobra — Wrong

➜

ॐ **Correlations with Yoga** ॐ

Sanskrit: *Bhujangasana* Variation
English: King Cobra Pose
Points: See *Bhujangasana*
Benefits: Stretches chest, shoulders, abdomen, and spine; strengthens spine and buttocks; alleviates asthma and sciatica
Contraindications: Back, neck, or wrist injury, pregnancy, headache

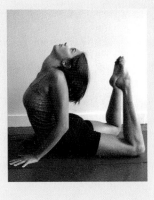

Advanced Variation: The King Cobra

The king cobra is an advanced stretch for more flexible clients. Bend the client's knees to 90° and sit on her extended feet. Make sure you have a steady seat before you pull her up.

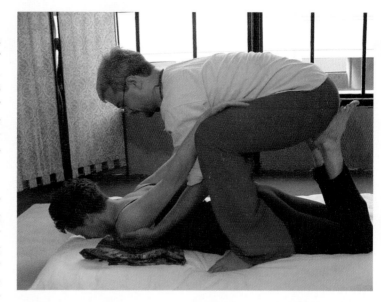

Next, take a hold of her shoulders by placing your hands through her armpits, and holding her deltoids with your palms. You can ask the client to place her hands on your legs (as shown in these photos), or have her leave her palms on the mat by her head if she is less flexible (as shown in yoga pose on previous page).

Using your feet to push off, lean back, placing your body weight into her feet while you lift her shoulders off the mat. Ask her to point her chin up towards the ceiling.

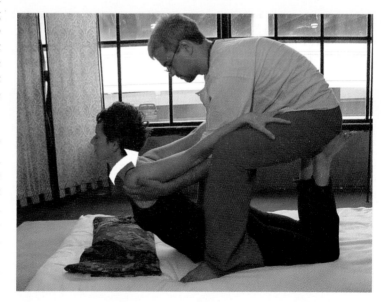

IMPORTANT: Your body weight through her legs should stabilize her pelvis and prevent her lumbar spine from taking the brunt of this stretch. However, if you see that the client's lower back is vulnerable in this position, skip this move.

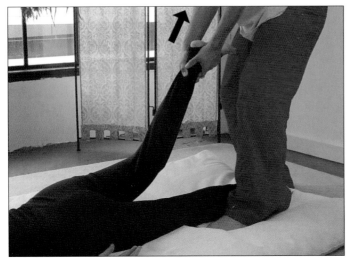

99. Single Leg Locust

Take hold of the client's ankle and lift by leaning back. This stretch targets the psoas and quadriceps. Be careful not to lift so high as to begin to stress her lower back. If her pelvis begins to lift off the mat, you have gone too far.

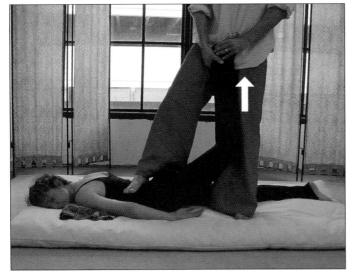

For someone who is more flexible, try the same stretch with your foot in her lower back.

Your foot applies light pressure to keep her pelvis square and firmly anchored on the mat. Be sure to place your foot on the soft part of her lower back, not directly on her spine or her pelvis. You can also try this step with light presses on her sacrum.

For a more flexible client, you can try this variation while lifting both her legs.

Repeat Step 99 for Other Side.

ॐ Correlations with Yoga ॐ

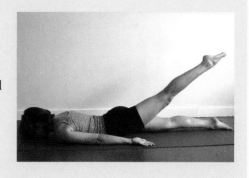

Sanskrit: *Ardha Salabhasana* Variation
English: Half-Locust Pose Variation
Points: Engage legs; tuck tailbone; lengthen spine
Benefits: Stretches quadriceps, hip flexors, and lower back; strengthens spine, buttocks, hamstrings and calves
Contraindications: Pregnancy, back or neck injury

ॐ Correlations with Yoga ॐ

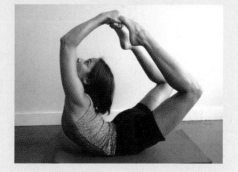

Sanskrit: *Dhanurasana*
English: Bow Pose
Points: Pull on ankles is very gentle to protect knees; inner thighs towards one another; tuck tailbone; spread collarbones and lift sternum
Benefits: Stretches spine, quadriceps, hip flexors, abdomen, shoulders, neck, and chest; strengthens legs, arms
Contraindications: Pregnancy, back or neck injury, high or low blood pressure, headache

**Variation for More
Flexible Clients**

For a deeper stretch in the single-leg locust, you can involve the client's arm as well. The top photo shows a lift on the same-side arm, while the bottom photo shows a lift of the opposite-side arm.

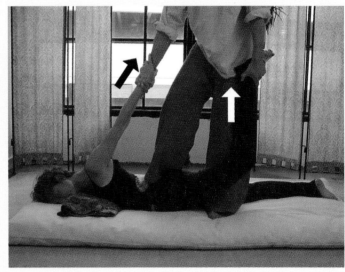

With either variation, it is important that you rotate the client's shoulder to open the chest before lifting, as with all back bends. Also, ask your client to turn her head in the direction of the arm which is being lifted, but to leave it relaxed on the mat during the lift.

Place your foot in her lower back on the same side as the arm you are lifting, and lift gently up through her leg and arm simultaneously.

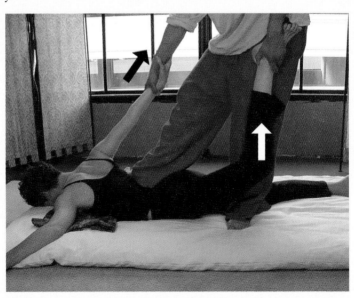

ॐ Correlations with Yoga ॐ

Sanskrit: *Natarajasana*
English: Dancer Pose
Points: This is an advanced pose and is not recommended without the guidance of a teacher
Benefits: Stretches the chest, shoulders, quadriceps, hip flexors, abdomen, spine, and neck; strengthens the feet, ankles, and legs; energizes spine and nervous system
Contraindications: High or low blood pressure; heart trouble; back, shoulder, neck or chest injury; headache, poor balance

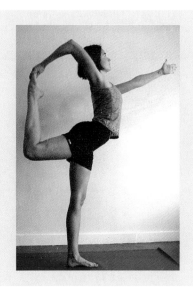

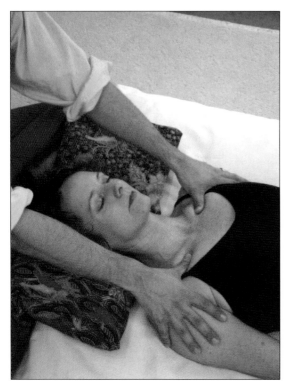

Head, Neck, and Face

100. Thumb Press Under Clavicles

Ask the client to turn over onto her back again and replace the pillow behind her head. Sit cross-legged behind her head so that you can work on the head and neck with the best body mechanics.

Note that this is the only time in a Thai massage that you should be above the client's head. When performing the classic routine, if you need to switch from one side of the client to the other, be sure to always walk around your client's feet instead of her head. The traditional reason for not walking round her head is that you will disturb the client's crown chakra. However, on a practical note, it is also a matter of safety since your client is on the floor. It's one thing if you trip over your client's feet as you walk by, but imagine if you accidentally kicked her head during a massage!

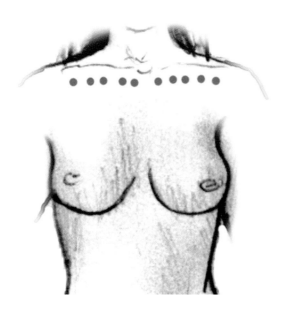

Our massage of the head, neck and face begins with thumb presses under the clavicles along the top of the pectoral muscles. Follow the line of the clavicles from the shoulders in toward the sternum, and then back out again.

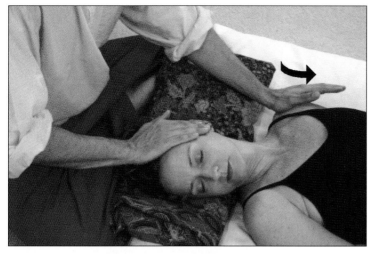

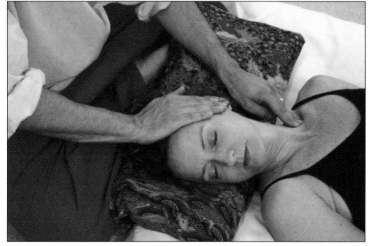

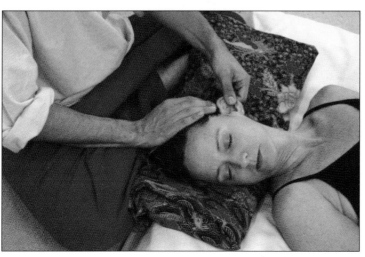

101. Gently Stretch Neck by Pressing on Shoulders

Turn the client's head gently to the side, keeping her neck straight. Place your hand on her head without adding any pressure. The stretch comes from pushing her shoulder away from her neck. Press the shoulder down into the mat and away from her ear.

Release the shoulder but continue to hold her head to the side. Gently use finger presses above the clavicles along the base of the neck muscles. Use a thumb on clients who enjoy more pressure. Follow the line of the clavicle laterally to medially. When you arrive at the midline, press gently into the sternoclavicular notch before moving back out laterally again.

Finish by finger circling up the side of her throat to the ear.

102. Ear Massage

Gently roll the ear lobe in between your thumb and fingers. Massage the entire ear, giving it a little tug in all directions. There are numerous acupressure and acupuncture points here, so be sure to stimulate the whole ear.

Gently roll her head to the other side, keeping the head straight.

Repeat 101-102 for the other side.

103. Finger Press Along Trapezius and Neck

Gently roll the client's head back to a neutral position. Apply finger presses along the trapezius muscle, working from the top of the scapulas to the spine and back out again. Use finger presses from below to gently lift her shoulders off the mat. You can also apply stronger thumb pressure into the trapezius muscles and at the base of the neck for clients who are particularly stiff. Press both sides at the same time, or use a walking motion.

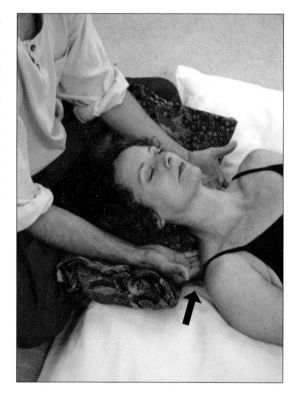

Next, we will continue the **back lines 1** and **2** up the neck. For **line 1**, as in the back, press gently between each vertebra. Use a gentle lifting with your fingers as you move up the neck and back down. **Line 2** is an inch or so out to the sides. Follow the neck muscles up to the base of the skull and back down again.

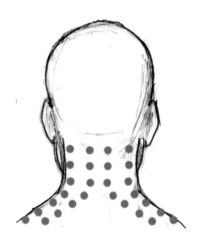

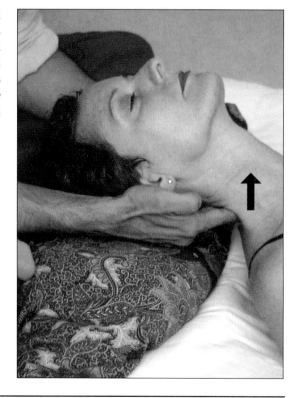

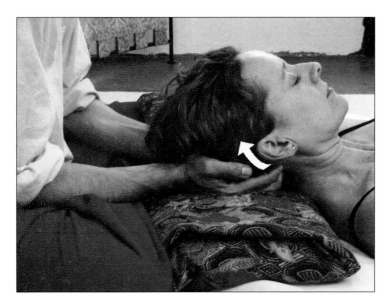

104. Base of Skull and Back of Head

At the base of the skull, hook your fingers into the points shown on the diagram below. Start laterally, and move towards the central point. Lean back and apply a little bit of pressure to the base of the skull by pulling towards you. Remember to use good body mechanics, rocking from your hips, not pulling with your arms. You are providing stimulus to the acupressure points while giving traction to the neck at the same time.

Next, gently walk with finger presses or finger circles up the lines shown in the diagram from the base of the skull to the temples. Finish by finger circling the temples.

Then, follow the middle line with finger and thumb presses from the base of the skull to the third eye, the point between the eyebrows. The client's head may roll gently from side to side as you walk your fingers up the back of the skull. Finish by circling the third eye with your fingers.

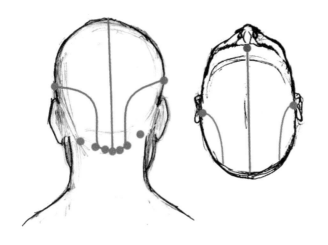

105. Forehead and Chin Lines

Follow the chin lines in the diagram below, moving from bottom to top. Begin in the center of the chin, and glide your hands outward towards the ears. End just under the ears at the TMJ with finger circles. Begin again at the midline, and repeat this motion. Each time, move your hands a little further up towards the mouth, so you cover the entire area, including the neck, under the jaw, and under the mouth.

Next, run your thumbs along the forehead lines. Begin at the third eye, and glide your thumbs along the eyebrows to the temples. Finish with gentle thumb circles on the temples. Move up a bit and begin again at the center. Keep repeating, each time moving up a thumb's width or so until you reach the hairline. Your last line should follow the hairline from the midline to the temples (shown in photo).

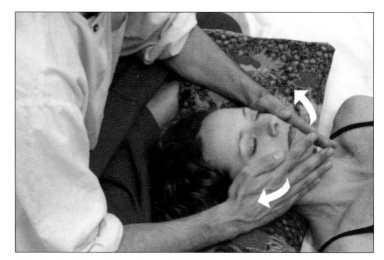

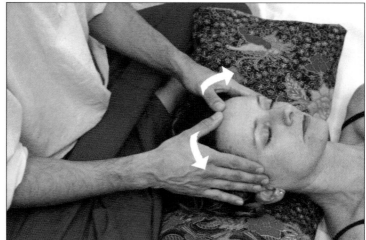

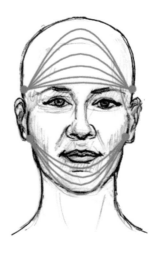

106. Scrub Scalp with "Shampooing" Motion

We have moved through the entire body from the feet to the head, and now we will finish the massage at the highest point on the body, the crown. This is traditionally seen in Thailand as the most sacred part of the body, as it is believed that our connection to the spiritual energy of the universe is via the crown chakra.

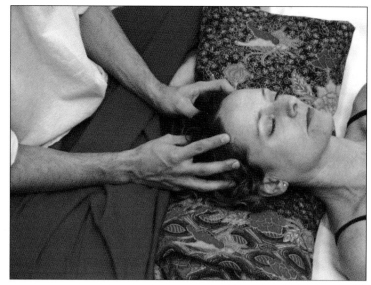

Use a scrubbing, "shampooing" motion all over the scalp. Turn the client's head to the side in order to access the whole head. Visualize that, having brought the energy up through the meridians throughout the course of the massage, you are now pulling out negativities through the crown.

107. Create a Vacuum with the Ears

The massage ends by allowing the client to go inside herself. Gently cup your relaxed palms around her ears. Create a vacuum by pressing inward toward the head (you may need to circle your hands a bit in order to make a tight seal).

Shut out from external stimulus, your client will travel inside herself, hearing only the sound of her own breathing, and perhaps her heartbeat.

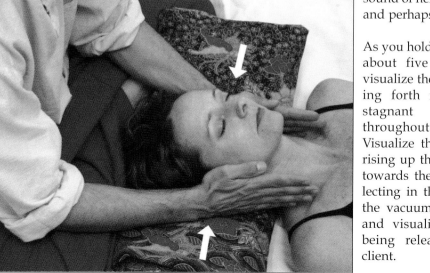

As you hold the vacuum for about five deep breaths, visualize the vacuum drawing forth impurities and stagnant energy from throughout the body. Visualize these negativities rising up through the body towards the head, and collecting in the ears. Release the vacuum with a "pop," and visualize this energy being released from the client.

108. Finish with a Prayer of Thanksgiving and Healing

Now that you have pulled out the negative energy, take a moment to fill your client with the beneficial vibrations of *metta*. Repeat mentally to yourself: "May you be happy. May you be well. May you be peaceful. May you be healed." Or, use your own affirmations.

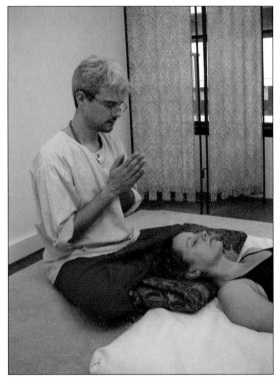

Traditionally, this is also a prayer of thanksgiving to the Father Doctor for the healing energies he has brought to you throughout the massage. The Thai therapist also will thank the client for her hard work by greeting the client when she opens her eyes with the "wai" gesture (shown in the photo) .

IMPORTANT: Don't omit this final part of the massage! Truth be told, this gift of *metta* may be the most important step of all. The entire massage routine can be seen from one perspective as an elaborate process to open the energy meridians of clients to enable them to receive this gift of healing and blessings from you at the end.

Allow your client a few minutes in silence. As she slowly emerges from her relaxed state, you may wish to assist her up into the seated posture. Try these steps from the classic routine to help her get up and moving again:

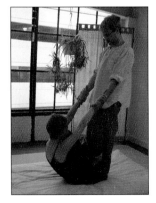

Cross-Legged Pull-Up

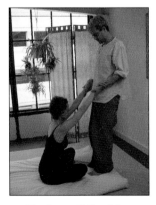

To Seated Position

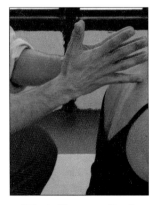

Thai Chop on Back

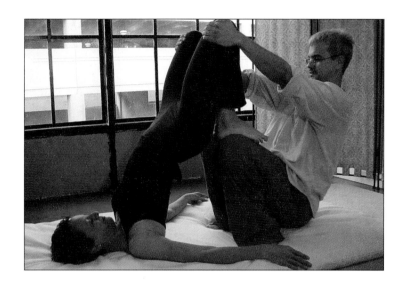

Chapter 5
Variations and Advanced Steps

This chapter will present some variations and advanced steps which you may wish to incorporate into your classic routine once you are familiar with the 108 steps introduced in Chapter 4. Use these steps as you see fit, keeping in mind clients' limitations.

Variations for Side Position

The side position variation is a routine you may wish to include in your classic Thai massage instead of the section for the back. You would typically use the side position for clients who are not comfortable lying on their front due to whatever reason (for example, pregnancy, obesity, or large chest). This routine also will play a role in the therapeutic massage introduced in Chapter 8, so you may wish to familiarize yourself with it before continuing.

The routine should be performed in the order presented, from beginning to end, as a substitute for the classic routine Steps number 78 to 99. Your client should then turn over and you should repeat the same steps for the other side of the body. Remember to start on the left side for a female client and the right side for a male client. Since you should already be familiar with the classic routine, detailed instructions will not be given in this section. Numerical references will be made to the classic routine, however, to orient you. Refer back to Chapter 4 for more information on each step.

For all of the steps in this section, the client is lying on her side, with her bottom leg straight and her top leg bent. A pillow or bolster under the bent leg may help to keep her sacrum perpendicular to the mat, which is desirable. Also, be sure that her shoulders are straight and that she has adequate support under her head to keep her neck straight.

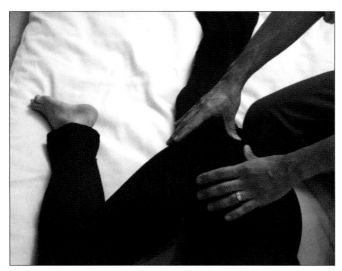

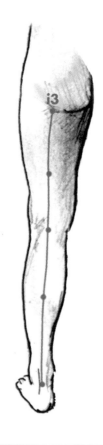

1. Foot Points and Leg lines
As with the classic routine for the back, you begin this section by pressing the foot points on the client's bent leg foot with palm presses and thumb circles.

From the foot, proceed with walking palm presses up her bent leg to the hip and then back down. Apply thumb presses along line i3, walking from the foot to the hip and back down again. Finish by repeating the palm presses.

(Compare to Steps 78-82.)

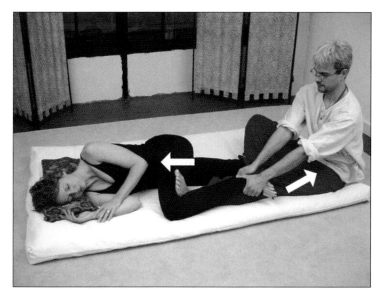

2. "Paddleboat"

Keeping the client's leg at a 90° angle, walk along line i3 with your feet, pressing into the back of her thigh along the hamstring from the knee to the hip and back.

(Compare to Step 19.)

3. Foot Press

Use your shin to keep the client's leg in the "figure 4" position while your feet press against the center of her hamstring. Reach out in front of you, and grab along lines i1 and o1. Pull towards you by leaning your body weight back. Pull five times.

(Compare to Step 20.)

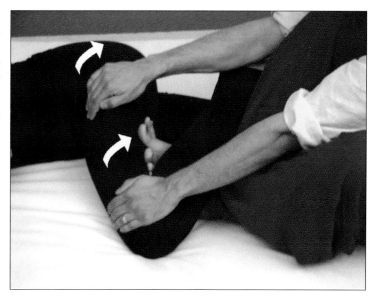

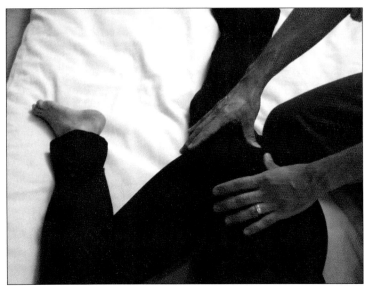

4. Hip Points

Press the points around the femur and below the iliac crest with thumb presses or, if your client prefers deep pressure, with elbow presses. Thumb press or circle the sacrum and glutes as well.

(Compare to Steps 88-90.)

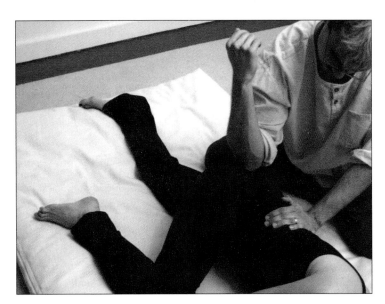

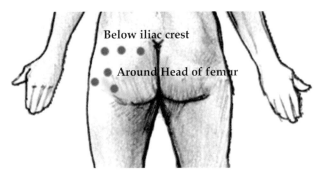

Below iliac crest

Around Head of femur

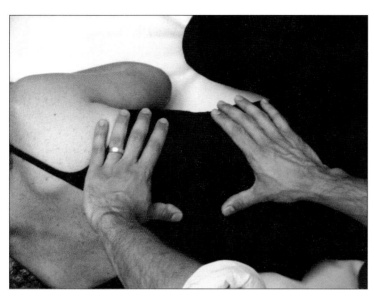

5. Back Lines

Begin the A-B-C-B-A pattern by placing one of your hands at the client's lower back and the other hand on her scapula, stretching her back. Next, palm press from the iliac crest to the scapula and back. Then, run along the three back lines with thumb presses. Finish the A-B-C-B-A pattern by repeating the palm press and stretch.

Note we will be working on only one side of the back for this step.

Finish by palm circling the client's rib cage from the scapula down to the waist.

(Compare to Steps 91-94.)

6. Shoulder mobilization

Bring your client's hand behind her back. Position your hands as shown in the photo on the right. Simultaneously pull her shoulder up and towards you while pressing with a bladed hand behind the scapula into the rhomboids.

From this position, you can also press behind the scapula with thumb presses.

(Compare to Steps 96-97.)

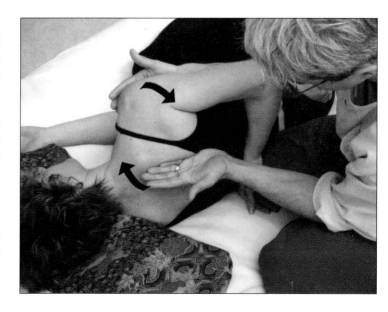

7. Triceps Stretch

Place the client's palm flat on the mat behind her ear so that her fingers are pointing towards her shoulder. Palm press her triceps to bring her elbow closer to the ground. From this position, thumb press along line o1 from the shoulder to the elbow and back again. Finish with another palm press.

(Compare to Step 48.)

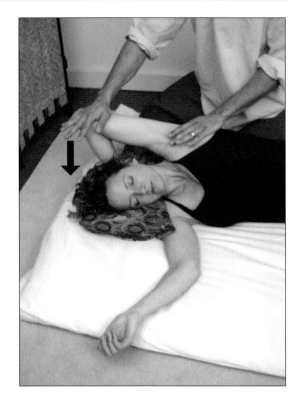

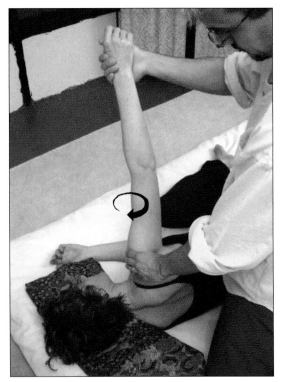

8. Rotate Shoulder and Pull Arm

Holding her wrist or hand with one of your hands, and stabilizing her shoulder with the other hand, rotate her arm five times clockwise and five times counterclockwise.

Next, pull her arm in all directions.

(Compare to Steps 42, 46.)

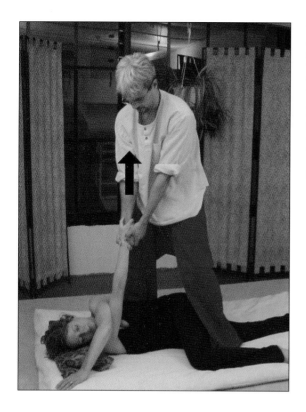

9. Arm Cross-Pull

Cross the client's arm over her body. Take her opposite arm under her crossed arm, and pull up to give a cross-stretch to her upper body, neck, and shoulder. Be sure you place the non-active arm between the stretching arm and the neck so as not to press into the client's throat.

(Compare to Step 47.)

10. Basic Back Stretch

Hook your forearm under the client's arm. Place your hand at her shoulder and your elbow in her lower back. Simultaneously press into your elbow while pulling back with your hand. This will provide a nice stretch for the back while preserving the opening in the shoulders that we look for with all back bends. Repeat three times with her exhalations.

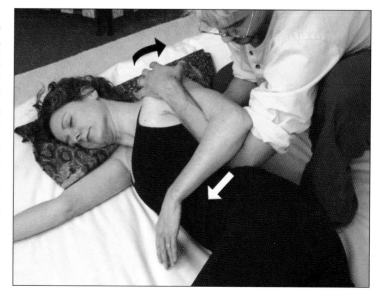

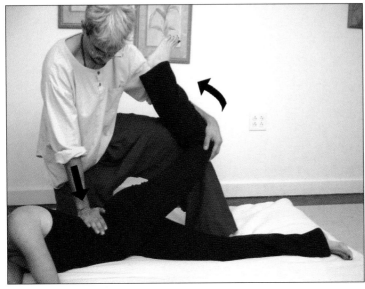

11. Locust Variations

Place the client's leg on your forearm, and take a hold on her knee. Apply your other palm to her lower back as shown in the photo. Shifting your body weight, pull her leg towards you while palm pressing into her lower back. This will stretch the quadriceps and psoas of the active leg.

If you find it more beneficial for your body mechanics, this same stretch can be achieved by using your knee in her lower back instead of your hand. Be sure not to knee press on the kidneys, rib cage, or other sensitive body parts.

(Compare to Step 99.)

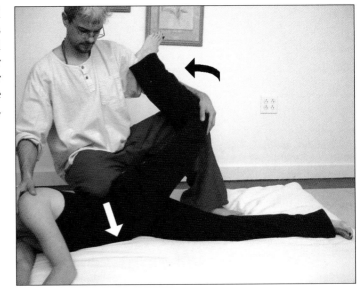

Advanced Variations

With a client who is a bit more flexible, there are two other options for performing this stretch. In the photo to the right, I am using my foot to apply pressure to the client's lower back, rolling her torso away from me, while I pull back on her ankle. This is a more intense version of the quadriceps/psoas stretch.

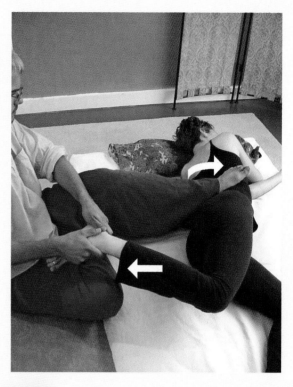

In the photo below, I am involving the back and shoulders more by holding onto the client's hand while performing the same stretch. If you use this variation, be sure to rotate the client's shoulder open as you do with all back bends.

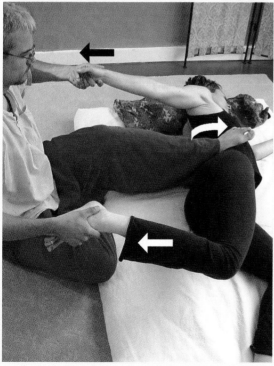

Variations for Seated Position

The seated position variations can be inserted either as a unit or individually into the classical routine at any point where the client is brought to a seated position. This can be done in the course of a 2- or 3-hour massage in order to extend the time, or it may be used as an alternative for clients who, for whatever reason, are not able to lie comfortably on the ground. (For example, clients with severe respiratory diseases or spastic diaphragms may prefer to remain seated throughout the massage). You may also find that these variations work well for chair massage. This series would make a great 15- or 20-minute demo massage for a client seated on an office chair or massage chair.

1. Thumb Press Back Lines
Begin by palm pressing along either side of the client's spine. Then, thumb press along all six back meridians (three on either side). Finish by palm pressing again. Remember to always work from the lower back to the trapezius and back down.

(Compare to Steps 91-94.)

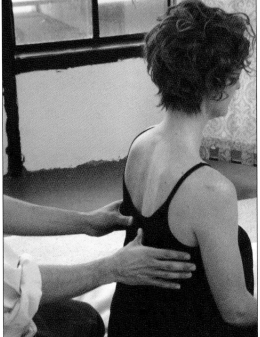

2. Scapula Mobilization
The scapula routine can be effectively performed from this position. Place your bladed hand against the rhomboids, and with your other hand rotate the client's shoulder up and towards you. Finish with thumb presses behind the scapula directly on the muscle.

(Compare to Steps 96-97.)

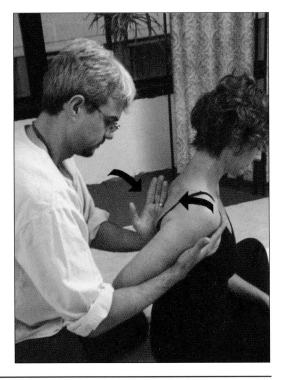

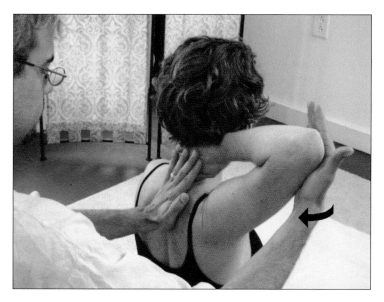

3. Triceps Routine

Place the client's hand on the back of her neck. Holding this hand in place, use your other hand to bring her elbow back towards you, stretching the triceps muscles.

Next, thumb press along line o1 from her shoulder to her elbow and back again.

(Compare to Step 48.)

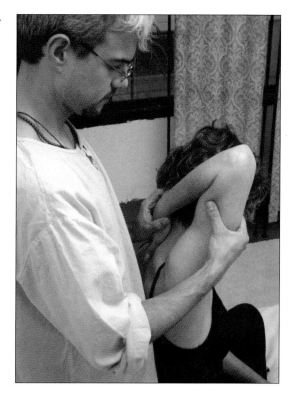

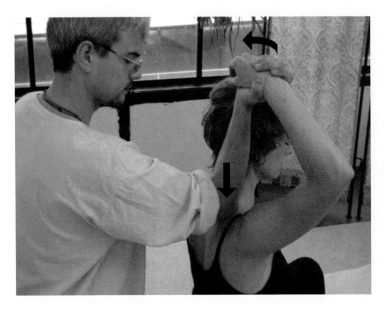

Alternate Method
For a client who enjoys more pressure, place your elbow on her trapezius muscle, and grip her wrist or hand. Pull her hand towards you to stretch the triceps muscles, while pressing your elbow into the trapezius muscle. This is a great combination of pressure and stretching.

4. Rotate Arm
Holding the client's wrist or hand in one of your hands and stabilizing her shoulder with the other, rotate her arm both clockwise and counterclockwise, five times in each direction.

(Compare to Step 42.)

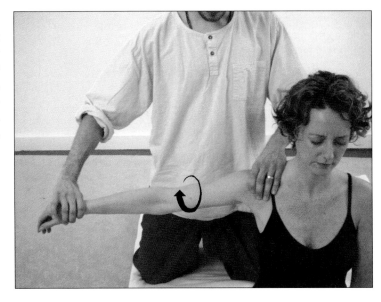

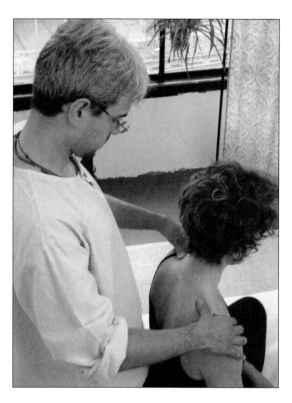

5. Thumb Press Trapezius

The trapezius is one of the most chronically over-worked muscles. Use body weight to thumb press down into the traps from above. Follow the lines shown in the diagram in Step 102.

(Compare to Step 102.)

6. Trapezius and Neck Stretch

In this step, you use your forearms to press the trapezius and shoulder down while pressing the neck to the side.

Place both of your forearms at the base of the client's neck. Applying a bit of pressure, roll your arms away from each other. Repeat this a few times.

IMPORTANT: Be sure always to press very gently when working with the neck.

(Compare to Step 101.)

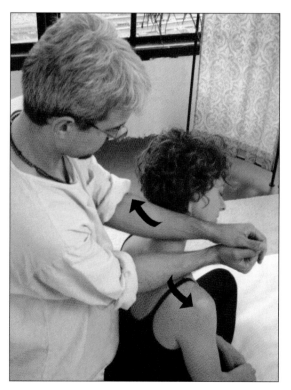

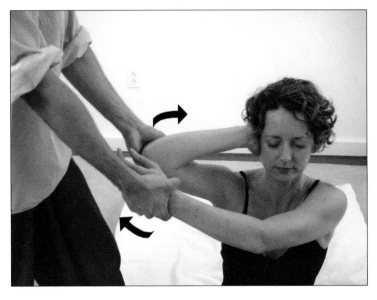

7. Advanced Neck Stretch

Place one of the client's hands on her ear. Cross her other arm in front of her torso and hold her wrist or hand. While pulling on this hand, press her bent elbow towards her head. This should cause her head to rotate as shown in the photo below, stretching the neck muscles. Perform this stretch smoothly with control in order not to strain the neck muscles.

This stretch can also be performed with your hand on the client's ear. The reason for using the client's own hand is that she will not permit you to overstretch her neck. A client would release her hand from her ear before the stretch became too intense. If you feel confident that you know your client and will not overstretch her, try this step using your own hand.

IMPORTANT: Be sure always to be sensitive to the client's abilities and limitations, especially when working with the neck.

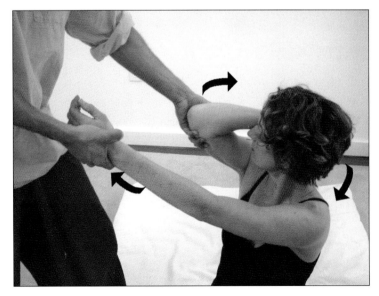

In Thailand, this step is often done very quickly as a chiropractic adjustment of the neck. Under no circumstances should this type of work be attempted by an untrained therapist.

8. Thumb Press Neck Points

Using thumb presses, follow the points shown in the diagram for Step 102. Follow both lines from the trapezius to the base of the skull.

Placing a palm on the client's forehead as shown in the photo to the right, you can assure that her head remains erect and her neck straight while applying this pressure.

Next, press upwards along the base of the skull points shown in the diagram for Step 103. Finish by following the three head lines from the base of the skull to the temples and the third eye.

(Compare to Steps 102-103.)

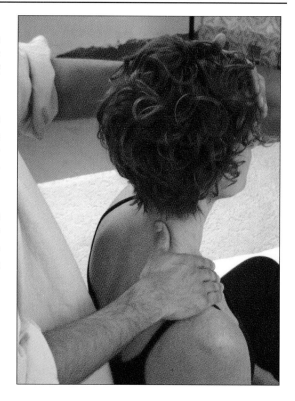

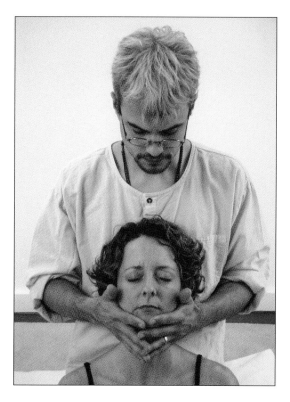

9. Face Massage

Rest the client's head against your chest. Perform the face routine as detailed in Step 105. Next, "shampoo" the scalp as shown in Step 106. Finish by stopping the ears as in Step 107.

(Compare to Steps 105-107.)

Advanced Stretches

After having finished reviewing the classic routine introduced in the Chapter 4, you may feel that Thai massage is a modality that is not for everyone. Certainly, there are clients who would be better off not receiving some of the more complicated yoga steps. These clients may prefer more concentration on meridian work (see Chapter 6), therapeutic routines (see Chapter 8), or herbal massage (see Chapter 9).

However, you will also find clients who enjoy the yogic postures, and who are ready for even more in-depth work than the classic steps. For these clients, you may wish to consider adding some of these more advanced moves.

The advanced techniques introduced in this section focus mainly on the back. They should be inserted into the classic routine in the appropriate place, during the yoga stretching section (or for the Full Locust, during the back section). Keep in mind, even with clients who prefer deep work and intense stretching, you should always warm them up with the classical routine steps such as thumb presses and light mobilization before attempting these advanced steps.

IMPORTANT: These advanced poses should not be performed by a therapist without adequate training and practice. These steps can potentially lead to injury for the client and/or the therapist when performed incorrectly. Proper understanding of alignment and body mechanics is essential at this level, and advanced training with a qualified instructor is highly recommended before attempting these steps.

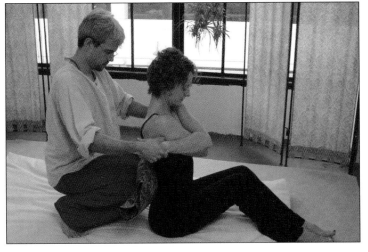

Advanced Back Stretch
This is a full back bend for more flexible clients only.

Begin by kneeling behind the client, and placing your knees just below her scapula. Use a cushion for padding.

Cross the client's arms in front of her, and take hold of her wrists.

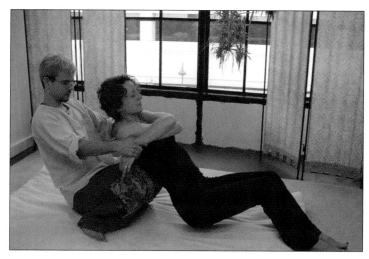

In one controlled and steady movement, lean back onto your heels and sit on the ground, bringing your client's pelvis off the mat. (When you are working with clients who are much heavier than you, it may be necessary to ask them to push off the ground in order to assist you in getting started.)

Let the momentum of your body weight continue to bring the client into a back stretch, over your knees. At this point, you should be completely relaxed, with your back fully on the ground.

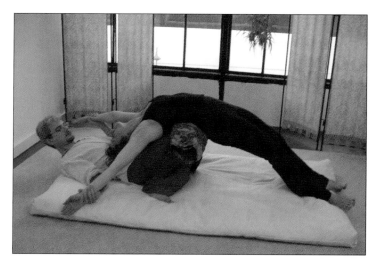

Unfold the client's arms, and bring them above her head. For an extra stretch, you can pull on her arms individually, or both at the same time. You could also hold her head and gently pull it towards you to give traction to her spine.

From this position, you can adjust the level of intensity of the stretch by raising or lowering your knees. Hold her in place over five breaths.

To release the posture, hold under the client's armpits. Simultaneously open your legs allowing her to slide between them, and lift her up into seated position.

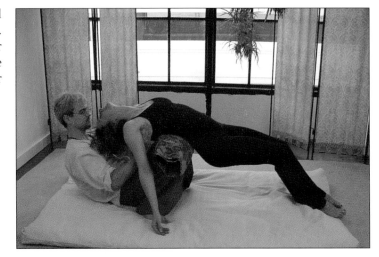

You should end in the same position in which you began.

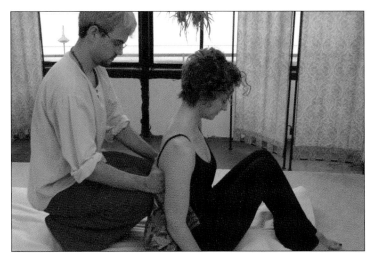

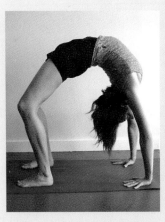

ॐ Correlations with Yoga ॐ

Sanskrit: *Urdhva Dhanurasana*
English: Upward Bow Pose
Points: This is an advanced pose. Outer edges of feet parallel, place hands so fingers point towards shoulders and elbows point towards ceiling; lift evenly using hands and feet, tucking tailbone and lifting sternum to open chest
Benefits: Stretches spine, quadriceps, hip flexors, abdomen, shoulders, neck, and chest; strengthens legs, arms and wrists
Contraindications: Back or neck injury, weak upper body, high or low blood pressure, headache

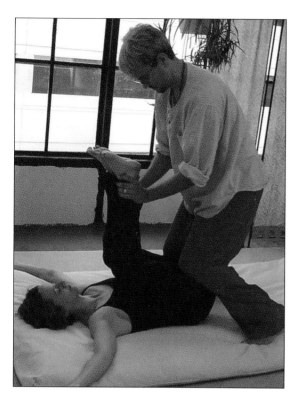

Bridge Pose

This is another wonderful back stretch, although it may be a bit harder to perform than the last one. You will have to experiment before attempting it on clients.

Begin by placing your knees in the hamstring insertions, at the very top of the back of the client's thigh.

Bring your client's legs towards you, and allow her feet to either rest on your hips, or open up to either side. Sit down while continuing to pull her legs towards you. Her hips should raise off the ground.

Hold this pose over five deep breaths.

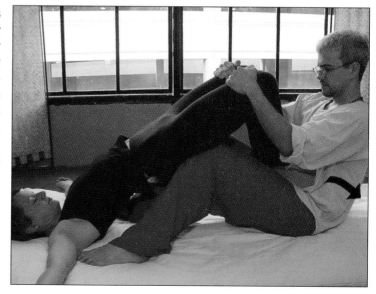

With more flexible clients, you can position your knees in the lower back so as to provide an even deeper stretch. (You may need to use a pillow to pad your knees.)

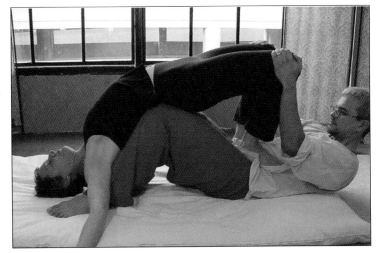

Release the client by unbending your knees.

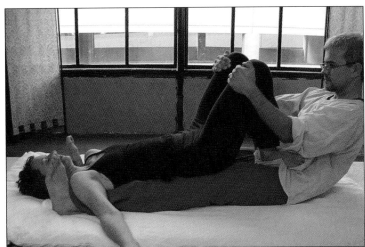

ॐ Correlations with Yoga ॐ

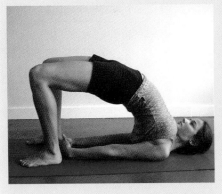

Sanskrit: *Setu Bandha Sarvangasana*
English: Bridge Pose
Points: Back of head remains on floor; outer edges of feet parallel; neck long; lift pelvis; tuck tailbone; lift sternum
Benefits: Stretches spine, chest, and neck; improves digestion; relieves asthma and sinus problems; relieves menstrual discomfort, mild backache, headache, insomnia; alleviates anxiety, stress and depression by calming nervous system
Contraindications: Neck injury, shoulder injury

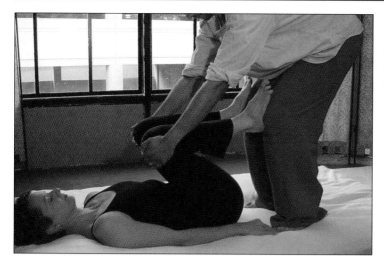

Shoulder Stand

This pose is the most difficult of the back stretches. Place the client's feet on your knees.

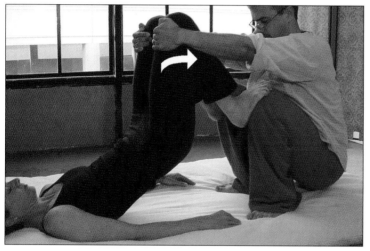

Keeping her knees together, sit back, and pull her pelvis off the ground.

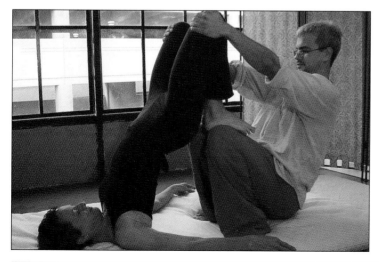

Lift the client up onto her shoulders, and hold this position for five deep breaths.

Release by retracing the steps you took to get into the pose.

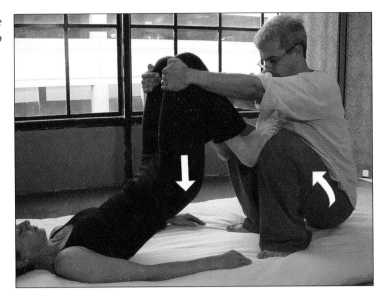

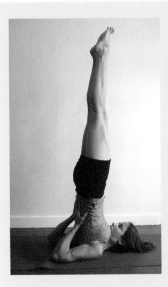

🕉 **Correlations with Yoga** 🕉

Sanskrit: *Salamba Sarvangasana*
English: Supported Shoulder Stand
Points: This is an advanced pose. Most easily approached from *Halasana* (Plow Pose). From *Halasana*, place hands next to spine with fingertips pointing up. Keep chest open as you lift legs.
Benefits: Stretches neck and shoulders; strengthens legs and back; improves asthma and sinusitis; alleviates stress, mild depression, fatigue and insomnia by balancing nervous system; stimulates thyroid, thymus, and prostate glands
Contraindications: Heart problems, pregnancy (if not part of regular practice), menstruation, high blood pressure, neck or spine injury, headache, diarrhea

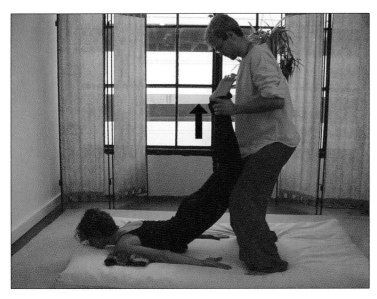

Full Locust

This is a very intense back stretch for flexible clients only. Begin by placing both of the client's legs together on the mat, and holding onto the client's ankles. Bring both of her legs up together so that her knees rest on yours (shown in the photo to the left). Your knees should be bent here so that you are supporting the client's weight with your legs rather than with your upper body or back.

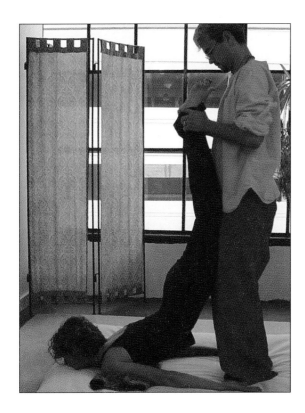

From this position, straighten your legs out to raise your client into the full locust. Walk forward a step or two if she can stretch this far. With an extraordinarily flexible client, you can ask her to bend her knees and bring her feet down toward her head, as shown in the yoga pose on the next page. (The ideal for this posture is to touch the floor in front of the head.) Hold this posture for five deep breaths.

Be very careful in this position that your client's lower back and neck are not overexerted. You can keep the pillow in its place under her chest in order to lessen the strain on her neck. Also, be sure to instruct your client to keep her chin on the mat, and her head straight. Under no circumstances should the client move her head or neck in this position.

To come out of the posture, retrace your steps. Take a step backward, bend your knees, place her knees on yours, and gently lower her legs back to the mat.

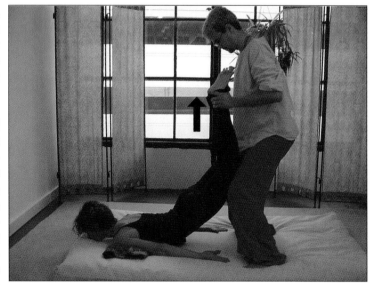

IMPORTANT: This is one of the most intense back stretches from the yoga tradition, and it should only be attempted with your most flexible clients. Be sure to provide the client with adequate lift throughout this step. If you do not continually lift her legs up towards the ceiling (even while lowering her down), her back will collapse, and her lumbar vertebrae will be stressed, potentially causing injury.

ॐ **Correlations with Yoga** ॐ

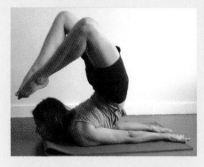

Sanskrit: *Salabhasana*
English: Full Locust Pose
Points: This is an advanced pose and is not recommended without the guidance of a teacher.
Benefits: Stretches the chest, shoulders, quadriceps, hip flexors, abdomen, spine, and neck; strengthens arms, legs, and spine; energizes spine and nervous system
Contraindications: Pregnancy; heart trouble; high or low blood pressure; spine, neck or shoulder injury

Walking Massage

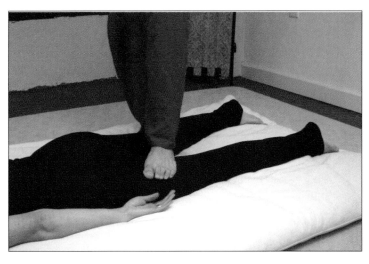

For clients who enjoy deep work, you can always use the knee press, foot press, or heel press to work the meridians or acupressure points throughout the body.

On the next few pages, I will introduce the technique of walking on the client's back, which is the most intense of the methods of applying pressure, and which should only be attempted with certain clients who enjoy a truly deep massage.

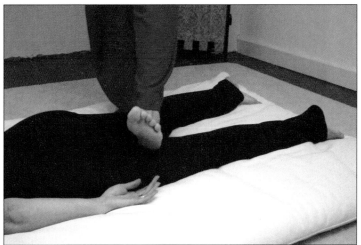

In Thailand, many practitioners have a rope suspended from the ceiling which is used for stabilizing the therapist during the back-walking. The therapist hangs from the rope for balance, while applying full body weight to the client.

In practice, this type of setup is not always possible in the modern massage clinic. A great alternative is to use a chair, stool, or other small piece of furniture for support. With practice, you may find that you are able to perform these techniques with no support at all, but you should reserve attempting this until you are fully competent with the steps outlined here so as not to slip and injure your client.

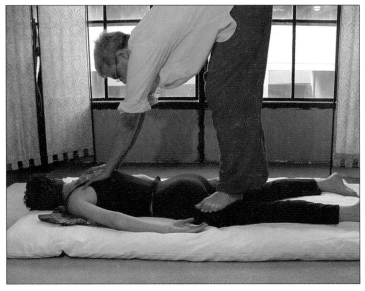

Standing Palm Press
To begin, stand on your client's thighs. Place both of your feet just under her buttocks, at the insertion of the hamstrings. This is a part of the body which can take a lot of pressure, and you probably won't hurt your client. If at this point your client feels pain, suspend further back walking steps and go back to thumb, palm, and elbow pressure.

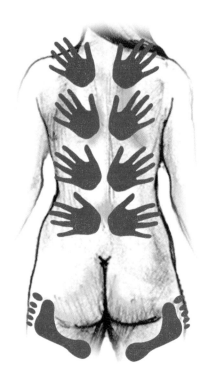

If your client enjoys this amount of pressure, apply your hands in butterfly palm position to the client's back. Remembering to always start from the lower back and work upwards, place a palm on either side of her spine, and press simultaneously with both hands. Move your hands up a palm-width, and press again. Press all the way up to the top of the scapula, being sure not to press directly on bone, and then work your way back down.

Never press the back in a jerky, quick way. Always use firm, steady application of pressure. Don't be surprised if the vertebrae crack during this step, but don't make this your goal.

IMPORTANT: For all of the steps in this section, never press directly on the spine!

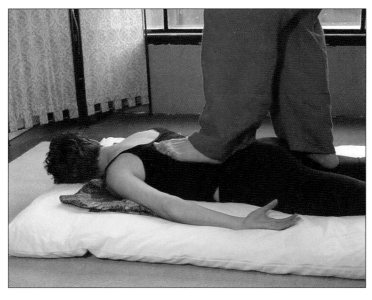

Walking on Back with One Foot

Keeping one of your feet stationary on the client's thigh, place your other foot on the client's glutes. Shift your weight fully into this foot, pressing down evenly through your foot while the client exhales. Shifting back into your stationary foot, release the pressure while your client inhales.

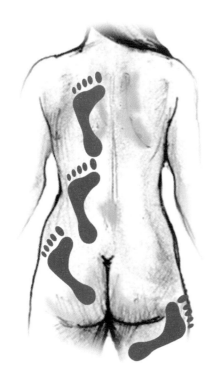

Move your pressing foot up to her lower back. Shifting your weight, apply another press. Repeating these motions, move your foot up the side of her spine, making sure you always press on muscle rather than bone.

Do not press higher than her scapula, as this would compromise the neck. Also, note how in the diagram, the positioning of your pressing foot changes with the contour of her back. With the press to the glutes, your foot is rotated outward to cover the entire buttock. However, with the presses on her back, your toes are pointed forward to apply weight evenly along the back muscles, and not directly on the rib cage.

If your client wants even more pressure than the foot press, you can repeat these steps with a heel press. (Be sure you keep your balance as you perform the heel presses!)

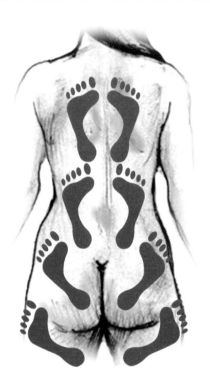

Walking on Back with Two Feet
When you have applied foot presses with one foot, try foot presses with both feet. This is the maximum amount of pressure you can apply to a client, with your full body weight directly on her back. Walk up on either side of the spine, as shown in the diagram to the left. Walk very slowly and deliberately, applying your weight in an even, controlled, and balanced manner. Remember to walk in synchronization with the client's breathing.

IMPORTANT: Be sure not to step on the spine, or to step higher than the top of the scapula to protect the neck!

Foot Press on Trapezius and Rhomboids
When you have completed the above steps, move around to stand at the client's head. Apply your foot to the client's back so that your heel is at the trapezius, and the rest of your foot lands between the scapula and the spine. Apply a foot press to this area. Move your foot if necessary to cover the entire trapezius and rhomboids.

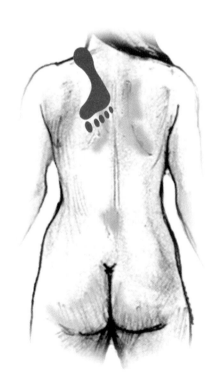

Note that in the diagram, I'm using my left foot to press on her left side so that the arch of my foot follows the contour of her scapula, minimizing the likelihood of stepping directly on the bone.

Part 2

Thai Yoga Massage Therapy

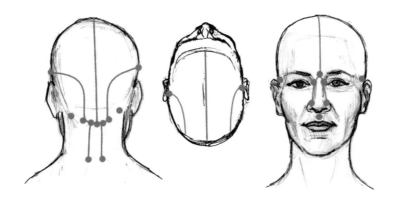

Chapter 6
Sen: The Thai Energy Meridians

Sen Lines

Although at first glance there seems to be some similarity between the Thai and the Chinese meridian systems, they are in fact quite different. The *sen*, like the Ayurvedic *nadis*, do not correlate, for example, with any organ systems the way that the Chinese meridians do. The Thai meridians all begin at the navel and end at the extremities of the body. Rather than corresponding to a single organ, the Thai meridians may be used to treat any and all organ systems through which they pass along their course.

The Thai *sen* share many similarities with their Indian counterparts, the *nadis*, and some even share the same names. For example, the *Sen Sumana, Sen Itha,* and *Sen Pingala* of the Thai tradition relate to the *Sushumna Nadi, Ida Nadi,* and *Pingala Nadi* of the yoga

tradition. The acupressure points used in Thai massage also are often identical to the Indian *marma* points. Even so, these two traditions are not interchangeable.

The Thai texts mention red, black, and white *sen,* which correlate roughly with arteries, veins, and nerves. However, traditional Thailand does not have a developed science of anatomy, and these distinctions are not generally very clear. Anatomy seems to play a minimal role in mapping the *sen. Sen* lines for the most part follow the grooves in between muscles, running along the insertion points. However, the same lines also take sudden turns into the body and are often difficult to trace exactly. Since the *sen* lines are not anatomically verifiable, and because of differences between Northern and Southern lineages, there are inconsistencies between schools across Thailand.

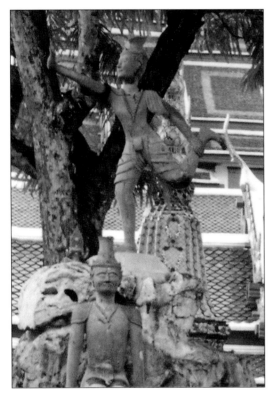

**Statues of figures in yoga postures,
Wat Po, Bangkok**

tions, it is technically incorrect. In this book, correlations with yoga and/or Chinese medicine will be pointed out when this is helpful to the practitioner, but the Thai system is introduced on its merits, as it is taught today in Chiang Mai. The descriptions of the 10 basic *sen* used in this book are based on the Northern lineage model, as taught by the Traditional Medicine Hospital of Chiang Mai.

Even if they do not agree exactly where the *sen* run, most Thai sources agree on names and symptoms associated with each *sen*. However, you may notice differences in spelling the *sen* from one book to the next. This is due to the fact that the academic community has remained undecided about a definitive method of transliteration for the Thai language. This means that as common a word as "hello" has been written in many different ways, including for example, *sawadi*, *sawatdee*, and *sawasdii*. In transliterating Thai, the Thais themselves are the most lax of all, interchanging *g* with *k*, *l* with *r*, and *d* with *t*. So, don't be surprised if you see *Kalatharee* spelled as *Galadhari*, or if you see *Itha* as *Eeda*.

The result of this confusion is that Western books on Thai tradition often differ slightly in their description of the *sen*. Although these differences are usually relatively minor, sometimes they directly contradict one another. Looking at three different books will often lead to three different maps of these meridians. This is simply because many of these writers have studied at different schools. A further confusion has been the effort on the part of some writers to combine different Asian traditions.

Because there are some similarities, many Western writers and teachers of Thai massage have mixed Thai with Indian or Chinese traditions when explaining massage techniques. While this exercise is useful to show the common origins of these medical tradi-

Under normal, healthy circumstances, the body's energy flows uninhibited throughout the 72,000 *sen* and is distributed according to the body's needs and activities. Problems arise in the body when these *sen* lines are either blocked or broken, causing an energy imbalance. (See Chapter 7.) Blockages and breaks are caused by a variety of reasons including sprains, muscle strains, injuries and stress. Parts of the body which are serviced by the *sen* lines can become affected by these energy imbalances and cease to function optimally.

The goal of *nuad boran* is to correct these energy imbalances by working directly with the *sen* lines to restore their vigor and vitality. Massage on a regular basis promotes healthy and strong *sen*, which fosters improved health and mental well-being. When a blockage or break occurs, therapeutic massage concentrates on restoring the body's normal function through stimulation of the affected *sen* lines.

For everyday Thai massage, it is helpful to view the body in terms of its individual parts rather than trace the *sen* lines directly. During a classic Thai massage routine, the practitioner moves throughout the body fully massaging each part before moving to the next. In this type of massage, the *sen* are not treated as individual wholes, but are massaged piecemeal as they are encountered. Thus, when the practitioner treats the legs of a client, for example, all *sen* of the legs are massaged, and when the arms are treated, all *sen* of the arms are massaged. In this way, the client is assured of a complete body massage, and all the main *sen* will be massaged, although not individually.

More advanced therapists will realize that the steps outlined in the classic routine provide a balanced massage precisely because they are continually cycling through the main *sen*, giving even attention to each.

On a theoretical level, however, it is important for the Thai therapist to understand each *sen* line as an integrated system in and of itself, an energy channel marked by particular acupressure points that enable the practitioner to manipulate the energy flow to certain limbs and organs. During a therapy routine, the practitioner will concentrate on an individual meridian and follow it on its course through the body. The diagrams beginning on the next page show the 10 main *sen* lines utilized in Thai massage therapy routines.

The *Sen*

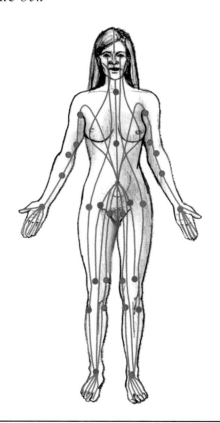

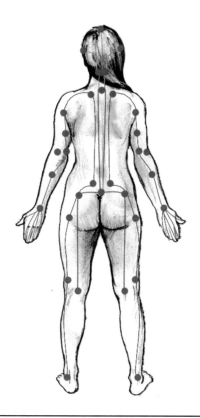

Itha & Pingala *Sen*

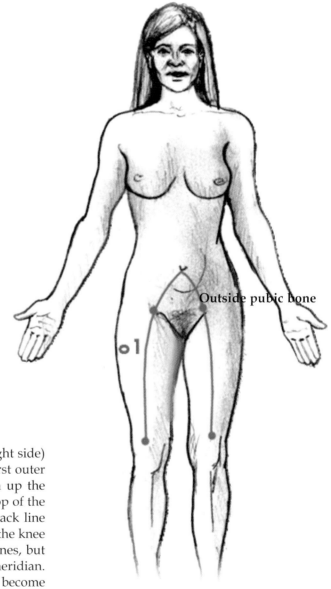

Outside pubic bone

o 1

The **Itha** (left side) and **Pingala** (right side) begin at the navel, run down the first outer leg line (o1), turn at the knee, run up the third inner leg line (i3), along the top of the iliac crest, and up along the first back line (1). The portion of o1 and i3 below the knee are considered secondary branch lines, but should be worked as part of this meridian. At the base of the skull, the two *sen* become three, with outer branches terminating at the temples, and the inner branch continuing over the top of the head, branching again at the third eye, and terminating at the nostrils.

The *Itha* and *Pingala sen* correlate to the back, knees, head, nose, and sinuses.

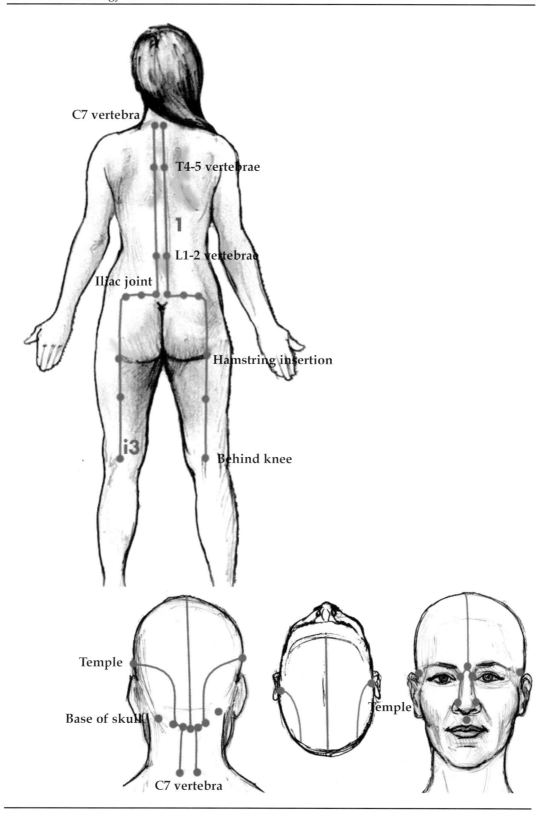

C7 vertebra

T4-5 vertebrae

1

L1-2 vertebrae

Iliac joint

Hamstring insertion

i3

Behind knee

Temple

Base of skull

C7 vertebra

Temple

Kalatharee Sen

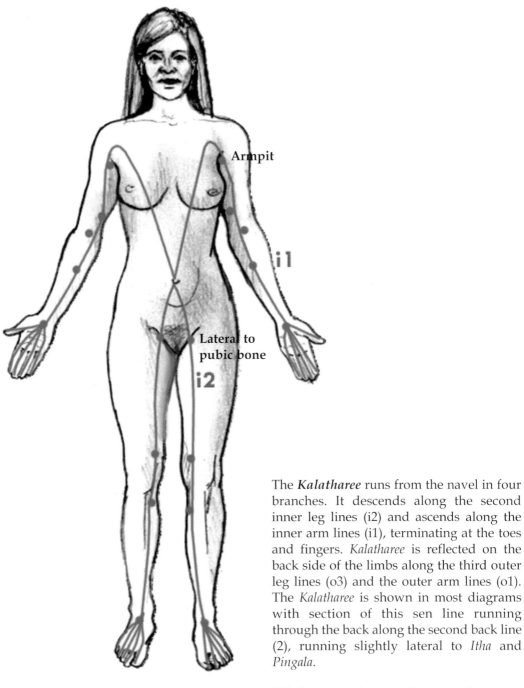

The **Kalatharee** runs from the navel in four branches. It descends along the second inner leg lines (i2) and ascends along the inner arm lines (i1), terminating at the toes and fingers. *Kalatharee* is reflected on the back side of the limbs along the third outer leg lines (o3) and the outer arm lines (o1). The *Kalatharee* is shown in most diagrams with section of this sen line running through the back along the second back line (2), running slightly lateral to *Itha* and *Pingala*.

Kalatharee correlates to the heart, chest, and limbs, as well as psychological and spiritual balance.

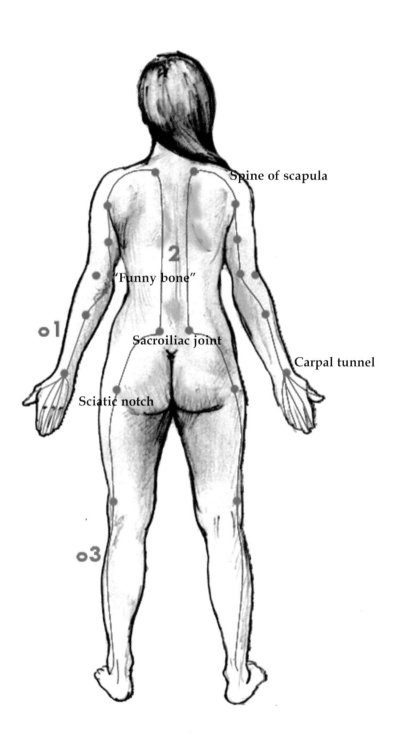

Spine of scapula

2

"Funny bone"

o1

Sacroiliac joint

Carpal tunnel

Sciatic notch

o3

Sahatsarangsi & Tawaree Sen

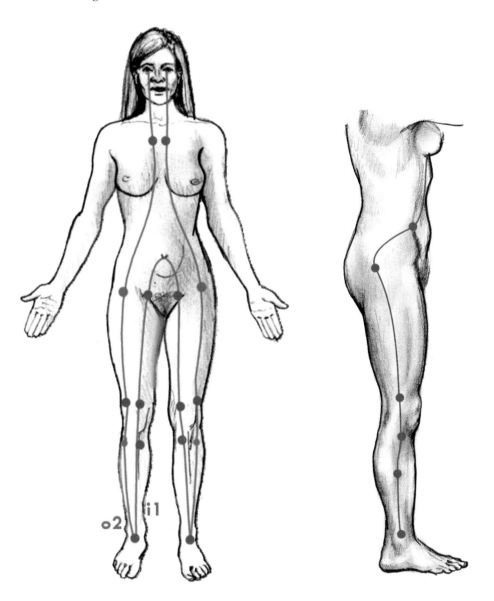

The *Sahatsarangsi* (left side) and *Tawaree* (right side) run from the navel, descend the first inner leg line (i1), turn at the ankle, ascend the second outer leg line (o2), and terminate at the eyes.

These *sen* correlate to the eyes, the lower abdominal region, and the chest.

Sumana Sen

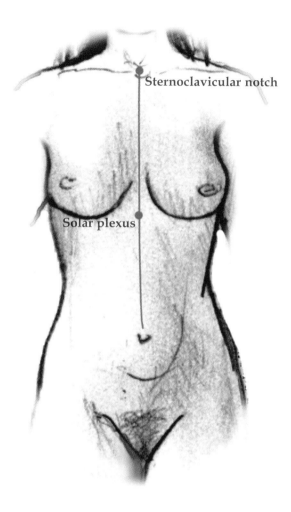

The **Sumana** runs from the navel to the base of the tongue.

The *Sumana* correlates to the upper digestive tract, heart, lungs, and upper respiratory system.

This *sen* approximately correlates to the *Sushumna nadi* from the yoga tradition, the meridian which runs up along the inside of the spinal cord and along which are found the six chakras, or main spiritual energy centers in the body. Thus, the *Sumana* is seen as a very important line of energy, and can be treated for most disorders.

Lawusang & Ulanga Sen

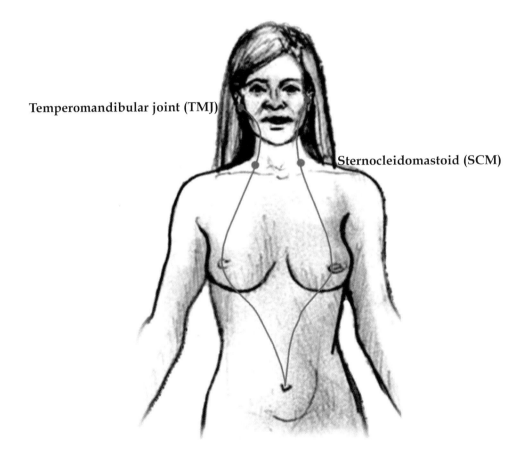

Temperomandibular joint (TMJ)

Sternocleidomastoid (SCM)

The *Lawusang* (left side) and *Ulanga* (right side) run from the navel, through the nipple, up the side of the neck, and terminate just below the ears.

These *sen* correlate to the breasts, ears, throat, mouth, teeth, and jaw.

Nantakawat & Kitcha Sen

The **Nantakawat** runs from the navel to the excretion organs in 2 parallel branches. The *Sikhinee* runs to the urethra, and the *Sukumand* runs to the anus. Abdominal acupressure points are discussed in more detail in Chapter 7.

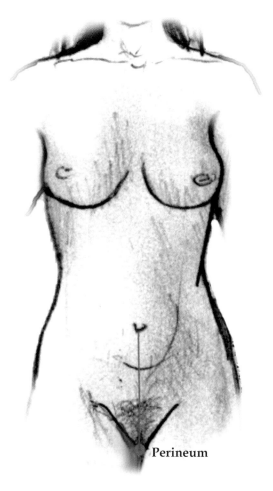

Perineum

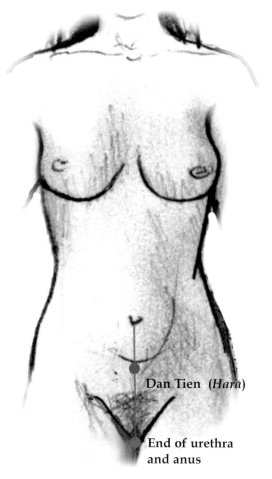

Dan Tien (*Hara*)

End of urethra and anus

The **Kitcha** runs from the navel to the perineum, passing through the reproductive organs. In the male, the *Kitcha* is called the *Pittakun*, and in the female, it is called the *Kitchana*. It correlates to sexual function and fertility, including the testes and prostate in men and the uterus and ovaries in women.

The perineum is the main acupressure point on this *sen*, but this point should not be treated with direct acupressure. It can be stimulated, with the patient's consent, by applying warm herbal compress.

Correlations between Symptoms and Sen Lines

Abdominal Pain/Disease/Disorders (Lower): Itha-Pingala, Kalatharee, Sahatsarangsi-Tawaree
Abdominal Pain/Disease/Disorders (Upper): Sumana
Acid Reflux: Sumana
Angina: Kalatharee
Anxiety: Itha-Pingala
Appendicitis: Sahatsarangsi-Tawaree
Arm Pain/Stiffness/Injury: Kalatharee
Arthritis (of limbs, digits): Kalatharee
Asthma: Sumana
Back Pain/Stiffness/Injury: Itha-Pingala
Bell's Palsy: Sahatsarangsi-Tawaree, Lawusang-Ulanga
Bipolar Disorder: Sahatsarangsi-Tawaree
Blood Pressure: Itha-Pingala
Breast Disease/Disorder/Cancer: Lawusang-Ulanga
Breathing, Difficulty of: Sumana
Bronchitis: Sumana
Cardiac Arrhythmia: Kalatharee
Cardiac Disease/Disorder: Kalatharee
Cataracts: Sahatsarangsi-Tawaree
Chest Pain: Kalatharee, Sahatsarangsi-Tawaree, Sumana, Lawusang-Ulanga
Chill: Itha-Pingala
Cold: Itha-Pingala, Sumana
Colon Pain/Disease/Disorders: Itha-Pingala, Kalatharee, Sahatsarangsi-Tawaree, Nantakawat
Constipation: Nantakawat
Cough: Itha-Pingala, Kalatharee, Sumana
Cramps, Menstrual: Nantakawat
Cramps, of Abdomen: Sahatsarangsi-Tawaree
Cramps, of Leg: Sahatsarangsi-Tawaree
Depression: Kalatharee
Diaphragm Spasm/Disorder: Sumana
Diarrhea: Nantakawat
Dizziness: Itha-Pingala
Ear Infection/Disease/Disorder: Lawusang-Ulanga
Epilepsy: Kalatharee

Erectile Dysfunction: Kitcha
Eye, infection of: Sahatsarangsi-Tawaree
Eyes: Itha-Pingala, Sahatsarangsi-Tawaree
Facial Paralysis: Sahatsarangsi-Tawaree, Lawusang-Ulanga
Fatigue: Itha-Pingala, Sahatsarangsi-Tawaree
Fever: Itha-Pingala, Sahatsarangsi-Tawaree
Finger Pain/Stiffness/Injury: Kalatharee
Foot Pain/Stiffness/Injury: Kalatharee
Gall Bladder Disease/Disorders: Itha-Pingala
Gastrointestinal Pain/Disease/Disorders (Lower): Itha-Pingala, Kalatharee, Sahatsarangsi-Tawaree, Nantakawat
Gastrointestinal Pain/Disease/Disorders (Upper): Sumana, Lawusang-Ulanga
Glaucoma: Sahatsarangsi-Tawaree
Gum disease: Sahatsarangsi-Tawaree
Hand Pain/Stiffness/Injury: Kalatharee
Headache: Itha-Pingala
Hearing Loss: Lawusang-Ulanga
Heart Disease: Kalatharee, Sumana
Hernia: Kalatharee, Sahatsarangsi-Tawaree, Kitcha
Incontinence: Nantakawat
Indigestion: Sumana
Infertility: Kitcha
Insomnia: Sahatsarangsi-Tawaree
Intestinal Disease/Disorders: Itha-Pingala, Kalatharee, Sahatsarangsi-Tawaree, Nantakawat
Jaundice: Kalatharee
Jaw Pain/Stiffness: Lawusang-Ulanga
Knee Pain/Stiffness/Injury: Itha-Pingala, Kalatharee, Sahatsarangsi-Tawaree
Lactation: Lawusang-Ulanga
Leg Pain/Stiffness/Injury: Kalatharee
Lethargy: Itha-Pingala, Sahatsarangsi-Tawaree
Liver Disease/Disorders: Pingala
Lungs Disease/Disorder/Infection: Sumana, Lawusang-Ulanga

(CONTINUED)
Menstruation, Irregularities or Pain: Nantakawat
Nasal Congestion: Itha-Pingala
Nausea: Sumana
Neck Pain/Stiffness/Injury: Itha-Pingala
Oral infection: Sahatsarangsi-Tawaree
Ovarian Disease/Disorder: Kitcha
Paralysis (of limb/s): Kalatharee
Paralysis (spinal cord injury): Itha-Pingala
Peptic Ulcer: Sumana
Prostate Disease/Disorder/Cancer: Kitcha
Psychological Disorders: Kalatharee
Reproductive System Disease/Disorder: Kitcha
Respiratory System Infection/Disease/Disorder: Sumana
Rheumatic Heart Disease: Kalatharee
Schizophrenia: Kalatharee
Septum: Itha-Pingala
Sex Drive, Lack of: Kitcha
Sexual Dysfunction: Kitcha
Shock: Kalatharee
Shoulder Pain/Stiffness: Itha-Pingala
Sinusitis: Itha-Pingala
Sore Throat: Itha-Pingala, Sahatsarangsi-Tawaree, Sumana, Lawusang-Ulanga

Stomach Pain/Disease/Disorder: Sumana, Lawusang-Ulanga
Stress: Itha-Pingala
Testicular Disease/Disorder: Kitcha
Throat Infection/Disease/Disorder: Itha-Pingala, Sahatsarangsi-Tawaree, Sumana, Lawusang-Ulanga
Tinnitis: Lawusang-Ulanga
TMJ: Lawusang-Ulanga
Toe Pain/Stiffness/Injury: Kalatharee
Toothache: Sahatsarangsi-Tawaree, Lawusang-Ulanga
Ulcer, Peptic: Sumana
Urinary Tract Infection: Itha-Pingala, Nantakawat
Urogenital Infection/Disease/Disorder: Itha-Pingala, Sahatsarangsi-Tawaree
Uterus Disease/Disorder: Nantakawat, Kitcha
Vaginal Infection/Disease/Disorder: Kitcha
Vertigo: Itha-Pingala
Vision, Impairment of: Itha-Pingala, Sahatsarangsi-Tawaree
Vomiting: Sumana
Weakness: Itha-Pingala, Sahatsarangsi-Tawaree
Whooping Cough: Kalatharee

The chart above points out correlations between symptoms and *sen* lines. To use this chart, locate the symptoms your client is exhibiting and determine which *sen* is affected. With this information you will be able to flip to the respective diagrams in this chapter and locate each *sen* as well as its corresponding acupressure points. Therapy routines for each *sen* line are discussed in Chapter 8.

Northern and Southern Styles

The most noticeable difference between the Northern and Southern lineages of Thailand can be seen in the manner in which the *sen* lines are manipulated. In the South of Thailand, centering around the Wat Po massage school, massage is almost always performed beginning at the navel and working outwards. In the North of Thailand, centering around the massage schools of Chiang Mai, a classic Thai massage always begins at the feet and ends at the head. Only in a therapy routine does the practitioner start at the navel, follow the *sen* out to the extremities, and then back again. Even then, this pattern is only followed for the 30-minute therapy routine, and then the feet to head pattern is resumed for the rest of the massage. (See Chapter 8 for more details on therapy routines.)

Another difference between these two lineages is the manner in which the *sen* are pressed. In the Northern style, practitioners follow a gentle technique of thumb pressing along the *sen*. Pressure is applied perpendicularly to the surface of the skin, pressing into the skin with increasing force, and then is slowly lifted off.

Southern style massage is a stronger form of manipulation. Practitioners still use the thumb press to apply pressure perpendicularly into the surface of the skin. Once the maximum force has been applied to the area, however, the practitioner quickly rolls the thumb across the *sen* line while lifting the thumb off. The resulting "zing" or "twang" delivered to the *sen* is sometimes a mild shock to the client, but when applied correctly is an effective method of relaxing tension, particularly in very stiff or sore muscles. With some practice, this technique can be an interesting and pleasant addition to the practitioner's repertoire of hand techniques.

To practice the Southern technique, and to test that the it is being performed properly, apply a "zing" to the middle of your forearm, along the inner *sen* branch. (See p. 33.) When this line is "zinged" correctly, the fingers of the hand should twitch involuntarily. Using this exercise as a guideline, practice applying the Southern style to other parts of the body. Note that this technique should not be attempted on clients without proficient practice. Additionally, great care must be taken not to dig into the client too hard, for more harm than good can result from improper use of this technique.

In their daily practice, many Thai therapists use Northern style for general full-body classic routines, and Southern style for the more intensive therapeutic routines for particularly stiff or sore areas. This should only be done if the practitioner is equally comfortable with both styles and can make a smooth transition between the two, as it is sometimes disconcerting to the client to change styles in the middle of a massage.

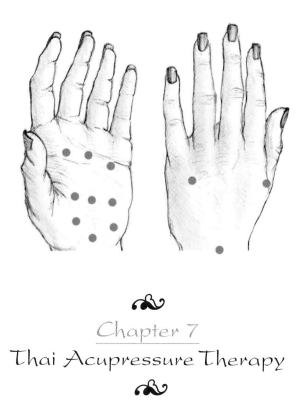

❧

Chapter 7

Thai Acupressure Therapy

❧

Acupressure Techniques

Thai acupressure, or *jap sen*, is an integral part of the practice of Thai therapeutic massage. The English word "acupressure" is used in modern parlance both as a name for a specific Chinese technique and as a more general term meaning simply pressure applied to particular points on the body. In this book, I always use the term acupressure in this more general sense. Thai acupressure, simply put, is the application of pressure (usually with the thumbs) to points that lie on a meridian, in order to stimulate energy. Pressure on these points is used to energize the meridian as a whole, and is an indispensible part of the therapeutic Thai massage routine.

Acupressure points frequently have a very different qualitative feel from the surrounding area. An acupressure point usually feels more sensitive, and often can hurt if pressed with more than mild pressure. Frequently, acupressure points can be found along major nerves, or next to bones or joints.

In this chapter I have presented an acupressure atlas of the human body, with diagrams of each of the common acupressure points used in Thai massage for therapy. These points are usually easy to find, and you can experiment on yourself until you get them right. Because these points are being pressed with a thumb rather than a needle, the therapist need not develop the detailed accuracy of the acupuncturist. However, it is important to find the correct point. Most times, if you begin with a thumb circle to help orient yourself, you will find the point with relative ease.

Three steps should be followed for application of acupressure to a point:

1. Before acupressure is applied to a point, the point should be warmed up with five clockwise and five counterclockwise thumb circles.

2. Acupressure should be given with thumb presses. Pressure should be applied with the ball of the thumb, perpendicularly to the surface of the skin. (See Chapter 3 for proper body mechanics for thumb press.) Each point should be pressed three times. Each time, the therapist should begin with slowly increasing pressure over a period of 5 seconds. Maximum pressure should be held for 2 or 3 seconds. The pressure should be lifted slowly over 2 or 3 seconds, for a total of about 10 seconds per point.

3. After acupressure, the point should be relaxed with five clockwise and five counterclockwise thumb circles.

It is important to note that only acupressure points should be pressed in the above manner. Never use acupressure on other parts of the body. Acupressure should never be administered to bones, "cold pressure" injuries (see below), or other sensitive areas of the body. Additionally, there are some acupressure points that are too vulnerable for thumb presses, such as the temples and many facial points. These can only be pressed gently with finger presses or finger circles.

Different body types will respond differently to acupressure, and the practitioner will have to practice in order to get a feel for "the right touch." As a general rule, larger, more overweight people are more sensitive to acupressure and require less pressure, although very thin people are also sensitive. Muscular people require more strength, and in extreme cases you may find it necessary to use elbow, knee, or foot presses to administer effective

stimulation. This is also true of clients experiencing paralysis or complete numbness. In these situations, maximum pressure is desirable, although care must be taken, of course, not to injure the client.

With any body type, pay careful attention to the client as acupressure is being administered. Over time, you will develop the ability to "hear" your client's body with your thumbs, and will never have to guess how much pressure is too much. For now, always start by giving less pressure than you think will be necessary, and build up if desired. Any twitch or grimace of the face, tightening or spasms of the muscles being touched, or other indication of discomfort from the client may be regarded as a sign to use less pressure. (Although in Thailand they would say, "No pain, no gain.") If the client is not comfortable, acupressure may have to be suspended. You may always use herbal compresses as a substitute for acupressure in sensitive clients. (See Chapter 9.)

Hot and Cold Pressure

Two major phenomena can occur to affect the sen lines negatively, breakage and blockage, and the knowledge of these conditions will determine how you apply acupressure. The difference between the breakage and blockage of a sen line is often difficult for the practitioner to perceive, as in both cases, the client will report pain as a symptom. It is important to differentiate between the two, however, since this will determine how you approach the meridian in question.

Breaks
The main causes of a *sen* break are muscle strains, tendon sprains, nerve pain, and bone injuries. *Sen* breaks are almost always acute conditions, brought on by a sudden injury, and need immediate attention. Broken *sen* lines cause energy to escape the channel and pool in the surrounding tissue. This is evi-

denced by swelling, redness, and sensitivity in the area.

These types of injuries typically produce sharp, shooting pain and are said to require "cold treatment." Herbal ice packs can be applied to the body part (see Chapter 9), and the massage practitioner should apply only indirect or "cold pressure" to this area.

Cold pressure is a technique to help dissipate pooled energy away from the affected area to allow the break to heal. Light thumb presses should be applied to the *sen* line above and below the break, and should move outwards, away from the affected area, all the way to the ends of the *sen* line or segment. At any time should the client experience pain, use a lighter touch. The practitioner should take care to never press directly on the site of the broken sen line, as this will cause an increase in pooled energy rather than contribute to its dissipation.

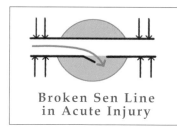

Broken Sen Line in Acute Injury

The diagram above shows a broken *sen* line with localized swelling (red). Black arrows indicate where pressure should be applied. Never apply pressure directly to the swollen area.

After 48 hours, a *sen* breakage will typically have begun to mend, and the swelling and heat will have subsided. At this point, cold therapy will give way to hot therapy, and the injury will be treated as a blockage in order to clear out stagnated energy and get things flowing again.

Blockages
Blocked *sen* lines are usually chronic condi-

tions caused by fatigue, stress, bad posture, and repetitive stress. Blockages usually manifest as muscle knots, tendonitis, localized stiffness, and soreness, but they can also be characterized by dull pain, weakness, stiffness, numbness, and sometimes even paralysis. Blockages are obstructions in the *sen* lines that cause the flow of energy to organs and limbs further along the channel to be inhibited, metaphorically analogous to cholesterol buildup in the arteries.

Sen blockages are treated with hot therapy: application of hot compresses (see Chapter 9), hot water baths, saunas, or "hot pressure." Hot pressure is direct acupressure on the location of the blockage with strong thumb presses to break up the obstruction and increase free flow of energy.

Some clients may require (or prefer) the use of the elbow, knee, or heel press on the site of a blockage, although care must be taken not to injure the client with these more aggressive techniques. *Sen* lines are particularly vulnerable at the site of a blockage, and too much pressure may cause a breakage. If a client is experiencing too much pain to effectively apply pressure to the blockage, hot compresses may be used instead (see Chapter 9).

Whatever method you use, be sure to apply strong presses to the site of the blockage, and then to move along the *sen* away from the site, as if "flushing" the blockage away. Travel all the way to the ends of the meridian or meridian segment, and finish by returning to the site. This encourages the disposal of stagnated energy, and then encourages the flow of fresh energy. Blockages also respond well to blood stops.

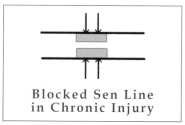

Blocked Sen Line in Chronic Injury

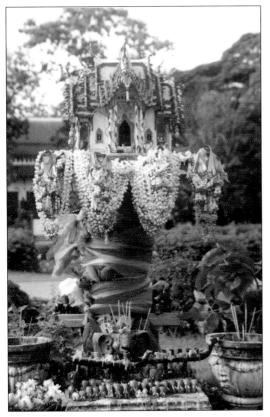

"Spirit House" altar in Chiang Mai with offerings of flowers and incense. (Note the lucky elephants in the foreground.)

The diagram on the previous page shows a blocked *sen* line. Arrows indicate where pressure should be applied, directly on the blockage.

Acupressure Atlas

I have found that virtually all of the points in the Thai system are also used in Chinese and/or Ayurvedic acupressure and acupuncture. (These points are known as *marmas* in India.) In the acupressure atlas which follows, I have drawn exclusively on the Thai tradition. However, because of the strong Chinese and Indian influence that permeated Thai medicine, you will see many parallels. The points in the hands and feet,

for example, are used to treat the entire body, as they are in Chinese reflexology. Readers interested in more information on Chinese or Ayurvedic acupressure or marmas should consult the bibliography for further reading suggestions.

These points are numbered in no particular order, and this numbering system is not a traditional one. I have simply numbered, in most cases, following from one extremity to the other. Until there is some agreed-upon system of numbering, the reader should not expect these numbers to correlate with those used by other schools or in other books. Note in the following diagrams that some points are shown in more than one picture to facilitate in locating them. Also note that points mirrored on the opposite side of the body are not numbered separately.

One final note, when working on a particular issue with acupressure, in addition to the points listed in the chart on the next page, the therapist should also press as many points as possible in and near the site of the problem. For example, the chart lists several points on the head for use in treatment of headache. These are simply the more effective points, but the therapist should not limit therapy to strictly these points. Other points in the head and neck should also be pressed. Likewise, because the *Itha* and *Pingala* are the *sen* lines most commonly associated with headaches, all of the acupressure points lying along both these meridians should be pressed. (Refer back to the *sen* charts in the previous chapter for these acupressure points.) Thus, acupressure for any particular disorder will cover the entire body.

Correlations Between Symptoms and Acupressure Points

Asthma: Hands 19, 22 Arms 5, 11 Torso 10, 13, 14, 15, 16, 17 Back 11, 15, 16, 19

Appendicitis: Feet 12

Back Pain/Injury/Arthritis: Feet 22 Hands 4, 22, 26, 30, 32 Legs 8, 28, 30, 31, 32, 33, 34 Back 1, 2, 3, 7, 8, 10, 11, 12, 13, 14, 15, 16, 18, 19

Breast Ailments: Torso 11, Back 15, 16, 19, 21

Breathing Difficulty: Hands 19, 22 Arms 5, 11 Torso 10, 13, 14, 15, 16, 17 Back 11, 15, 16, 19

Constipation: Feet 9, 10, 11, 12 Torso 2, 3, 4, 5, 6, 7, 8, 9, Head 9, 8

Cough: Hands 22, 36, 37, 38, 39 Arms 5, 11 Torso 10, 13 Back 11, 15, 16, 19

Dizziness: Head 10, 16

Ear Ailments: Hands 36, 37, 40, 41 Feet 1, 2 Torso 12 Head 5, 6, 7, 13

Erectile Dysfunction: Legs 1, 3, 4, 5, 7, 26 Arms 7 Torso 2 Back 9, 10 Head 19

Eye Ailments: Feet 3, 4 Hands 38, 39, 42, 43 Legs 7 Head 18

Facial Pain/Numbness/Paralysis: Hands 5 Head 5, 8, 9, 20

Fainting: Head 10, 16

Fatigue: Legs 26 Torso 5 Head 10, 16, 17, 19

Fever: Hands 34 Back 4

Gastrointestinal Ailments: Hands 4, 5, 8 Legs 8, 10 Torso 7, 8, 9, 10 Back 9, 10, 11, 15, 16, 19 Head 14

Headache: Feet 7 Legs 2 Hands 4, 5, 6, 9, 10, 11, 17, 20, 26 Head 2, 3, 4, 5, 6, 7, 12, 13, 17, 16, 19

Heart: Feet 7 Hands 17

Heel Pain/Injury: Legs 25, 27, 28

Hiccups: Torso 17

High Blood Pressure: Feet 7, 16 Hands 1, 5, 10 Arms 23 Back 10, 11, 17, 20, 21 Head 2, 3, 4, 19

Hip Pain/Injury/Arthritis: Legs 33 Hand 20, 26 Arm 14 Torso 2, 3 Back 8, 9, 10, 11

Indigestion: Feet 8 Hands 4, 5, 8 Legs 8, 10 Torso 7, 8, 9, 10 Back 9, 10, 11, 15, 16, 19

Infertility: Legs 1, 3, 4, 5, 7, 26 Arms 7 Torso 2 Back 9, 10 Head 19

Insomnia: Legs 10,21 Hands 17, Head 16

Kidney Ailments: Torso 6

Knee Pain/Injury/Arthritis: Legs 2, 6, 7, 8, 11, 12, 13, 14, 15, 16, 17, 19, 20, 22, 30, 31, 32

Leg Pain/Injury/Arthritis: Legs 3, 4, 5, 6, 8, 19, 20, 22, 23, 25, 26, 28, 29, 30, 31, 32 Arms 12, 15, 16, 23

Liver Ailments: Feet 6

Lungs: Hands 19, 22 Arms 5, 11 Torso 10, 13, 14, 15, 16, 17 Back 11, 15, 16, 19

Menstruation: Legs 1, 3, 4, 5, 6, 10, 25 Torso 6, 7, 8, 9, 20 Back 8, 10, 15, 16, 19 Head 19

Motion Sickness: Hand 24, 19 Arms 3

Mouth: Torso 14, 15, 16, 17 Back 17 Head 8, 9, 10, 12

Nausea: Hand 24, 19 Arms 3 Head 8

Neck Pain/Injury/Arthritis: Leg 6 Hand 2, 4, 5, 24, 32, 34 Arms 5 Torso 13 Back 20, 21, 22, 23, 24 Head 1, 2, 3, 4

PMS: Legs 1, 3, 4, 5, 6, 10, 25 Torso 6, 7, 8, 9, 20 Back 8, 10, 15, 16, 19 Head 19

Psychological Ailments: Head 16, 17

Reproductive System Ailments: Legs 1, 3, 4, 5, 6, 10, 25 Torso 6, 7, 8, 9, 20 Back 8, 10, 15, 16, 19 Head 19

Respiratory Ailments: Feet 7 Hands 28 Arms 5, 11 Torso 10, 13, 14, 15, 16, 17 Back 11, 15, 16, 19

Sacroiliac Joint Pain/Injury/Arthritis: Legs 33 Hand 20, 26 Arm 14 Torso 2, 3 Back 8, 9, 10, 11

Sciatica: Feet 15 Hands 6 Legs 3, 4, 5, 6, 8, 19, 20, 22, 23, 25, 26, 28, 29, 30, 31, 32 Arms 12, 15, 16, 22, 23

Sex Drive, Loss Of: Legs 1, 3, 4, 5, 7, 26 Arms 7 Torso 2 Back 9, 10 Head 19

Shoulder Pain/Injury/Arthritis: Hand 2, 3, 4, 6, 7, 8, 30, 31, 32, 33 Arm 17, 22, 23 Torso 13 Back 8, 17, 20, 21, 22, 23, 24 Head 1, 2, 3, 4

Sinuses: Head 3, 4, 9, 14

Sore Throat: Hands 34 Torso 10, 13

Stomach Ache: Hands 4, 5, 8 Legs 8, 10 Torso 7, 8, 9, 10 Back 9, 10, 11, 15, 16, 19

Stress: Feet 7, 16 Hands 1, 5, 10 Arms 23 Back 10, 11, 17, 20, 21 Head 2, 3, 4, 19

Toothache: Head 12 Hands 5, 7

Vomiting: Hand 24, 19 Arms 3 Head 8

Acupressure Points of the Feet

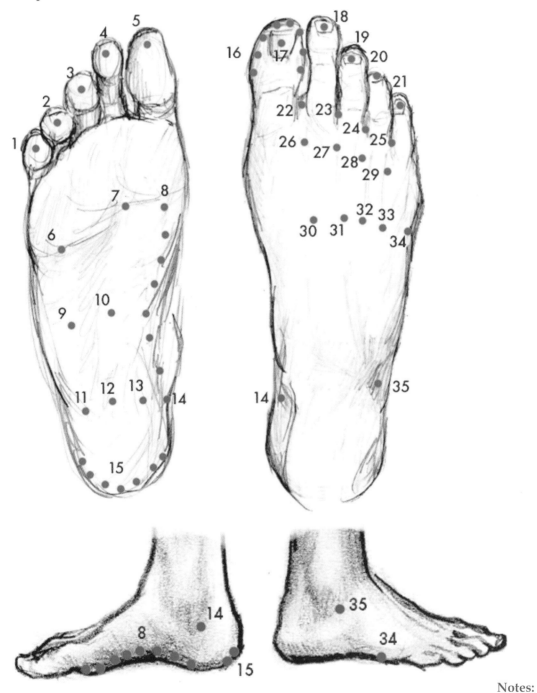

Notes:
8. Along the entire arch of the foot.
15. Include the entire perimeter of the heel.
16. Include the entire perimeter of the big toe.
22-33. Between the metatarsal bones.

Acupressure Points of the Hands

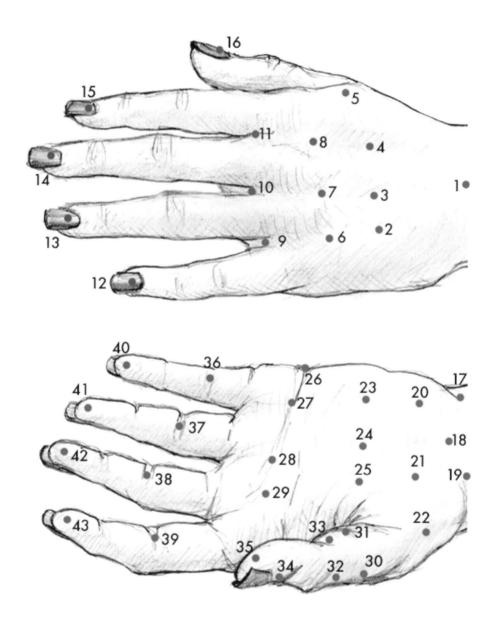

Notes:
2-11. Between the metacarpal bones

Acupressure Points of the Legs

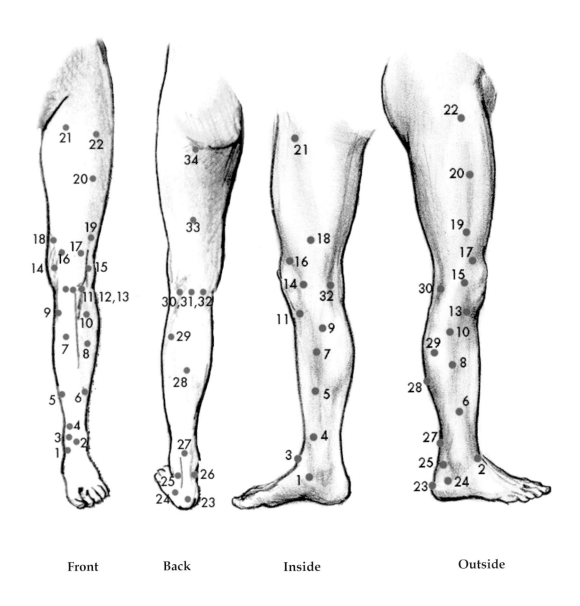

Front   Back   Inside   Outside

Notes:
21. Femoral blood stop point
11-16. Circumference of knee

Acupressure Points of the Arms

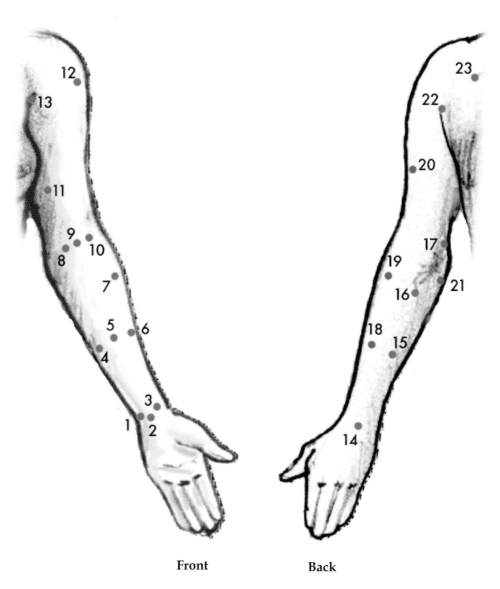

Front   **Back**

Notes:
8-10. Inside elbow
11. Brachial Plexus
13. Armpit
17. "Funny bone"

Acupressure Points of the Torso

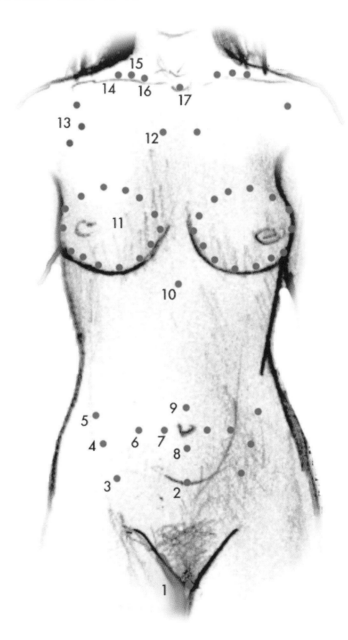

Notes:
1. Perineum
2. Dan tien (Hara)
3-5. Along the psoas muscle, inside of the hip bone
10. Solar plexus
11. The entire perimeter of the breast
13. The outline of the deltoids
17. Sternoclavicular notch

Acupressure Points of the Back

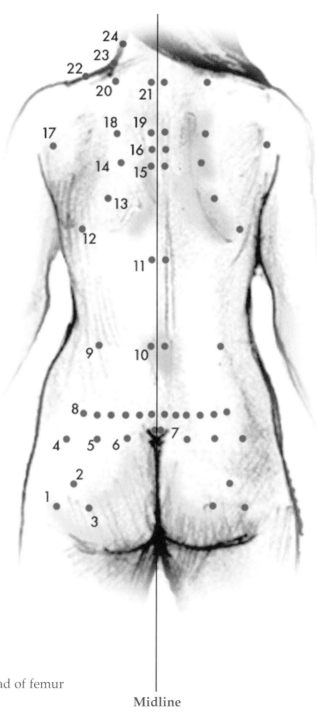

Notes:
1-3. Surrounding head of femur
4-6. Below iliac crest
7. Sacrum
8. Along iliac crest

Midline

Acupressure Points of the Head

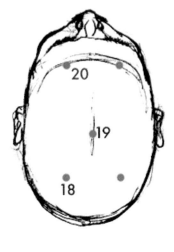

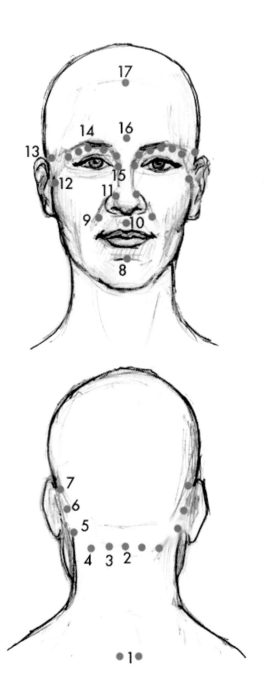

Notes:
1. C7 vertebra
2-5. Base of skull
11. Nasal passage
12. TMJ
13. Temple
14. Around eye orbit
16. "Third eye"

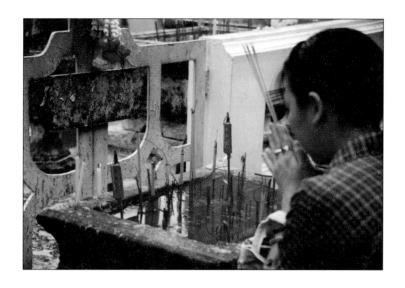

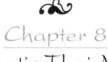

Chapter 8
Therapeutic Thai Massage

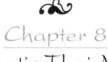

Sen Line Diagnosis

In Thailand, massage is a medical field and Thai massage therapists are trained in diagnostic arts. In the West, however, diagnosis is generally the realm of the professional physician, and massage therapists should tread lightly into this territory. In many areas, the word "diagnosis" itself is not permitted in the massage therapy setting.

Sen line diagnosis is a combination of experience, observation and intuition. It is a true art, and is often very difficult for a beginning therapist. Your powers of observation can guide you in the delivery of an effective massage, but never attempt to diagnose serious conditions without sufficient training. Always interview your client concerning specific symptoms, and ask if a professional

diagnosis has already been made.

Thai healers use a variety of tools for diagnosis — ranging from Chinese techniques such as tongue, iris, and pulse diagnosis to Ayurvedic methods such as the Four Elements. More often than not, however, traditional Thai healers are guided not by a specific system of diagnosis, but by intuition and the ability to "read" energy in their clients. Many masters of *nuad boran* are able to sense where the client's body is imbalanced merely by scanning or palpating the body, by working the meridians, or simply by observation.

Most Thai therapists use some combination of different techniques, but their diagnosis inevitably leads them towards an understanding of the imbalances in the individual client, and they design massage routines to assist in bringing back balance.

Often, a classic Thai massage routine such as presented in Chapter 4 can be the ideal way to bring balance back to a client. The routine is designed to treat all of the main 10 *sen*, to move energy through the body, and to purify it at the same time. However, with clients who present specific conditions, you may wish to add a therapeutic routine into the standard massage. This chapter will help you to design a therapy routine for a client based on the symptoms exhibited. Your first step is to diagnose the client's imbalance.

Thai Massage, *Tridosha*, and the Four Elements

One of the most common methods of diagnosis used in traditional Thai medicine is Four Element Diagnosis. This is a topic discussed in detail in my book, *A Thai Herbal*, so I will only briefly introduce it here. The Four Elements are the key to traditional Ayurvedic diagnosis, and are used by Thai herbalists to prescribe effective medicines. Thai massage therapists can also benefit from knowledge of these theories, since they can draw connections between diagnosis and *sen*.

The Four Elements describe the qualities of particular processes in the human organism, on the physiological, psychological, and spiritual levels. Each of the elements is associated with particular organs, emotional states, and *sen* lines, and using these correlations, a Thai therapist can gain a clearer picture of the type of therapy which will be most beneficial for a client. The chart on the next page can be used to draw connections between physiological, psychological, and spiritual symptoms and potentially blocked meridians.

Traditional massage therapists in Thailand do not typically use the Ayurvedic *tridosha* to diagnose and treat clients. Instead, they usually rely on more intuitive ways of "reading" their clients. However, *tridosha* may be a useful tool for the Western therapist who is already experienced with this basic Ayurvedic concept and is able to apply this knowledge to Thai massage. I am introducing this material here simply as a useful point of reference or comparison. The second chart on the next page provides a quick reference, drawing parallels between the *Doshas*, the Four Elements, and the *Sen*. (For more information and tools for evaluating a client's *dosha*, refer to the Further Reading at the end of this book.)

Once you have determined which *sen* line needs to be worked on, you can decide whether this line needs soothing (cold therapy) or stimulation (hot therapy). As a general rule, if you find one particular element to be excessive, work first to soothe the corresponding meridian. Then, focus on stimulating the meridians corresponding to the other elements. For example, if a client is excessively *Pitta*, or has an elevated fire element, you may wish to clear out the corresponding *sen* line, the *Pingala*, with cold therapy while working the other meridians to help the client back into balance. Conversely, a client with excessive *Kapha*, or earth element, might benefit from having the *Itha* cleared out with cold therapy while the fire element is stimulated by deep, Southern style work on the *Pingala*.

Sample Therapy Routines

Once you have determined the *sen* lines which are in need of treatment, you will design your therapeutic massage routine. A typical therapy routine is a 30-minute treatment of a particular *sen* line or lines, but the therapy routine may be of varying length,

Correlations between the Four Elements and the *Sen*

Element	Physical Processes	Psychological and Spiritual Processes	Corresponding *Sen*
Earth	Skin, muscle, bone, connective tissue, fat	Lethargy, fatigue, obesity, stagnation	*Itha*
Water	Blood, eyes, body fluids, urine, semen	Stagnation, stubbornness, rigidity	*Sahatsarangsi, Tawaree*
Air	Respiratory system, intestines, sexuality, aging, mobility of joints	Stress, anxiety, nervousness, inability to commit, fear, psychological disorders	*Kalatharee, Sumana, Lawusang, Ulanga, Nantakawat, Kitcha*
Fire	Body temperature, circulation, metabolism, infection	Aggression, tension, jealousy, violence, short temper, obsessive, overly sexual	*Pingala, Kalatharee*

Correlations between the Three Doshas and the Sen

Predominant *Dosha*	Element(s) in Excess	Corresponding *Sen*	Suggested Yoga Poses[7]
Kapha	Earth, Water	Itha	Cobra pose, hamstring stretches, headstand, plow pose
Vata	Air	*Kalatharee, Sumana*	Sitting variations, cobra pose, locust poses, forward bends, spinal twist
Pitta	Fire, Water	*Pingala*	Sitting variations, shoulder stand, fish pose, cobra pose, forward bends, spinal twists

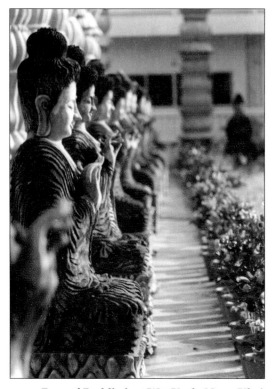

Row of Buddha's at Wat Kaek, Nong Khai

should be incorporated in such a way as to integrate it into the flow of the massage, while requiring the least amount of adjustment on the part of the client or the therapist.

Wherever it is inserted, it is important that the 30-minute therapy routine be performed without interruption, so it should not be mixed with classic routine steps. This is to ensure the integrity of the energy work. If you are stimulating a particular *sen*, and then start working with other parts of the body, you can inadvertently reverse the work you are performing.

One of the best solutions is to insert the therapy routine at the point in the massage where you are going to ask your clients to turn over onto their stomach or side. Before they make this adjustment, begin the therapy routine on the front side of the body. Then, ask them to turn. Continue the therapy routine on the back side of the body. When the therapy routine has been completed, return to the regular flow of the classic routine.

depending on the needs and condition of the client. Effective massage therapy balances concentration on the afflicted area with a concern for the harmony of the entire body. In Thai massage, a therapy routine is always incorporated into a whole body massage. This is to ensure that the affected areas are dealt with within the context of a balancing treatment for the entire body. The transition between full body massage and therapeutic routine should be seamless, and the client should never know where one begins and the other leaves off. (A general rule of thumb is to schedule at least 2 hours for a therapeutic massage. This is to ensure that you have enough time to provide a 1.5 hour classic routine and still be able to spend a good 30 minutes on the therapy.)

Where you choose to insert the therapy routine into the classic routine is up to you, and will depend on many factors. The therapy

The therapy routine will, in essence, follow the *sen* line or lines being worked from their origin at the navel to the ends and back again. The therapist will follow the meridian with thumb presses, or whatever method of pressure is most appropriate, and may stop to apply acupressure to points along the line as they are encountered. The therapy routine will also incorporate yoga postures from the classic routine in a specific order to additionally stimulate the *sen* line being worked. For example, a therapy routine on the *Itha* and *Pingala* lines will incorporate acupressure to the legs, back, neck, and face, as well as hamstring stretches, quadriceps stretches, and forward bends, because these all lie along the *sen* being treated.

In the interest of maintaining the harmony of the whole body, it is important to note that therapy routines are always performed symmetrically. Even if the injury or chronic condition occurs only on one side of the body, the exact same therapy routine is to be given to both sides of the body in order to preserve the balance of energy throughout the *sen*, and to address issues of "compensation" that may occur as the other side of the client's body tries to make up for the injured side.

The sample routines on the following pages contain numerical references to the classic and advanced steps presented in this book. These examples will help you to determine which steps to concentrate on during a therapeutic routine. Focus on these steps when giving the massage, repeating them more than once if you desire, and stimulate the acupressure points on the *sen* that run through the listed parts of the body.

When working with *sen* in a therapeutic massage, it is important that you remember to work the meridian from its beginning at the navel to its termination at the extremities. When referring to the steps listed on the following pages, you will often have to reverse the order of the instructions given in Chapters 4 and 5 in order to achieve flow in the desired direction. You should also remember to run over the *sen* line with thumb presses to connect the steps that you are performing.

Quick Reference: Correlations Between Sen and Treatment

Sen Affected	Suggested Yoga Postures	Suggested Acupressure
Itha & Pingala	Forward bends, hamstring stretches, plow pose	Knee, back, neck, head, and face
Kalatharee	Spinal twists, hip-openers such as hip adduction stretch, hip abduction stretch, "figure 4" stretch, arm stretches	Legs and arms, back
Sumana	Cobras and other back bends, spinal twist, all forward bends	Chest and throat, back
Sahatsarangsi & Tawaree	Stretches for iliopsoas, hips, cobra pose and other back bends	Neck and ears
Lawusang & Ulanga	Neck stretches, cobra and other back bends	Leg, face
Nantakawat	Spinal twists, forward bends	Stomach, abdomen
Kitcha	Gentle abdominal compressions, spinal twists, forward bends	Stomach, abdomen, hot compress on perineum

Therapy Routine for *Itha* & *Pingala*

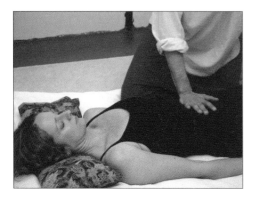

Palm Circles on Stomach (Step 55)
The *Itha* and *Pingala sen*, like all the Thai meridians, begin at the navel. Since we will be following the course of the sen through the body, we also begin here with a palm circle and press on the navel.

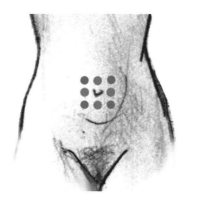

Thumb Press Stomach Points (Step 56)

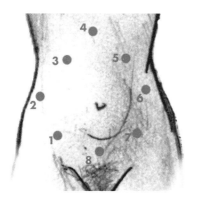

Palm Press Stomach Points (Step 57)
(Use any or all of the three options presented in Step 57.)

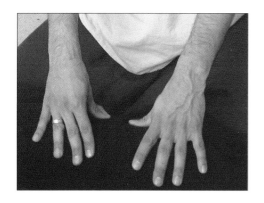

Work Meridian o1 and i3

Beginning with the appropriate side (left for *Itha*, right for *Pingala*), start this step with a stretch and palm press. Next, thumb press line o1 from the abdomen to the feet. Note that because you are working from the navel to the extremities, the direction is reversed from that of the classic routine.

When you reach the feet, turn and work your way up the back of the leg along line i3. You might find the side-lying position to be the most convenient for this step. Finish with palm press and stretch.

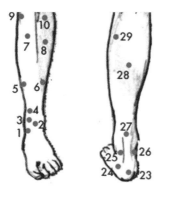

Acupressure of Leg

Refer back to the acupressure atlas and work with the following points: Legs 11, 12, 13, 16, 17, 31.

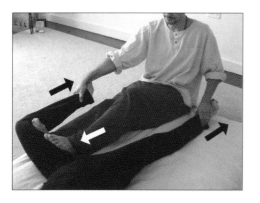

Foot Presses on Line i3 (Steps 19-21)

Still only working on one side of the body, press into i3 with feet and heels. This step can also be performed from the side-lying position.

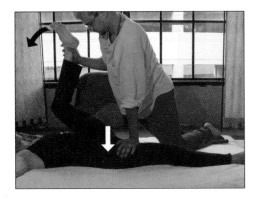

Hamstring Stretches (Steps 26, 32, 62, 63)
Do some or all of the hamstring stretches from the classic routine.

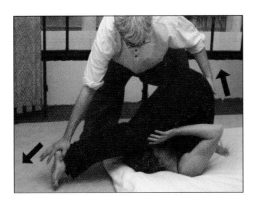

Plow (Step 65)
This pose engages the Itha and Pingala lines from the heels to the neck.

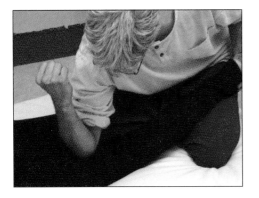

Elbow Press and Forearm Roll Line i3 (Steps 83–84)

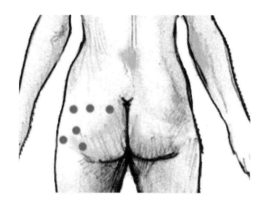

Acupressure of Hip (Side Position 4)

If you haven't already, switch your client to the side position shown in Chapter 5. From this position, press the acupressure points of the appropriate hip with thumb or elbow presses. Refer back to the acupressure atlas and work with the following points: Back 1, 2, 3, 4, 5, 6.

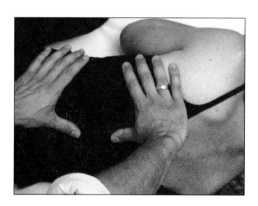

Back Meridians (Side Position 5)

With the client still in the side-lying position continue to work only on one side of the body; press along back line 1. Work from the lower back to the trapezius and back again.

Also, perform acupressure for the back. Refer back to the acupressure atlas and work with the following points: Back 8, 10, 11, 15, 16, 19, 21.

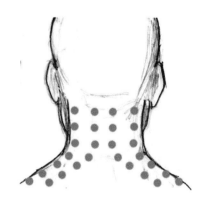

Trapezius and Neck
(Step 103)

Working only on one side, press from the shoulder up to the neck.

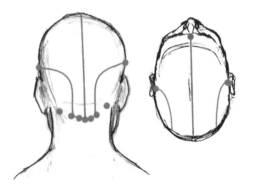

**Meridians and Acupressure of Head
(Step 104)**
Follow the *Itha* or the *Pingala*, whichever one you are working with, up to the temple, and over the crown to the nostril. Refer back to the acupressure atlas and work with the following points: Head 1, 2, 3, 10, 11, 16, 17, 20.

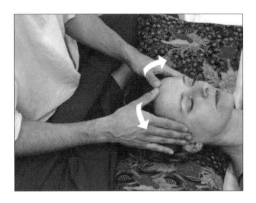

**Face Routine and Acupressure
(Steps 105-106)**
Refer back to the acupressure atlas and work with the following points: Head 10, 11, 16, 17.

Having followed the *Itha* or the *Pingala* from its origin to its terminus, reverse these steps to return to the navel. Then, repeat for the other side.

Therapy Routine for *Kalatharee*

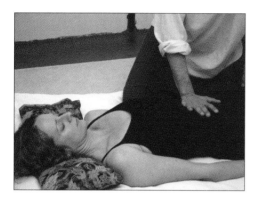

Palm Circles on Stomach (Step 55)
Begin at the navel with a palm circle and palm press.

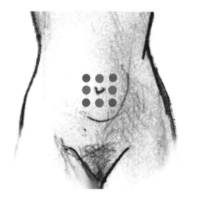

Thumb Press Stomach Points (Step 56)

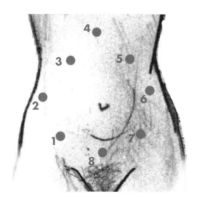

Palm Press Stomach Points (Step 57)
(Use any or all of the three options presented in Step 57.)

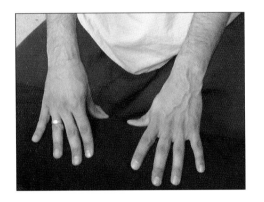

Work Meridians i2 and o3

Beginning with the appropriate side (left for female, right for male), start this step with a stretch and palm press. Next, thumb press line **i2** from the abdomen to the feet. Note that because you are working from the navel to the extremities, the direction is reversed from that of the classic routine.

Next, begin again at the hip and thumb press line **o3** down to the feet. Finish with palm press and stretch.

Acupressure of Leg

Refer back to the acupressure atlas and work with the following points: Legs 1, 3, 5, 9, 8, 18, 19, 20, 22 Back 1, 2, 3

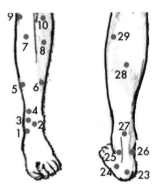

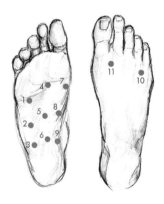

Foot Routine (Steps 2-7)

Still only working on one side, perform these steps for the foot.

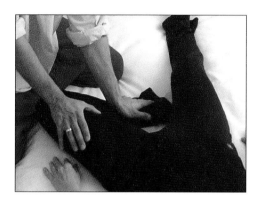

Figure 4 Hip Stretches (Steps 17-18)

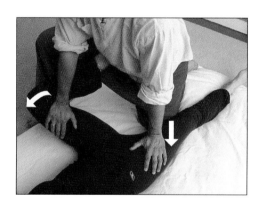

Lateral Hip Stretch (Step 27)

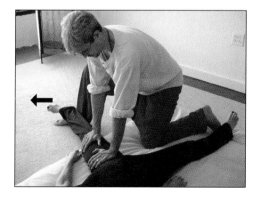

Abduction of Hip (Step 33)

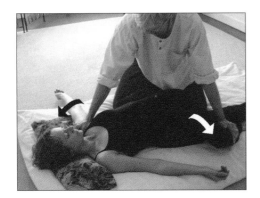

Spinal Twist (Step 28)

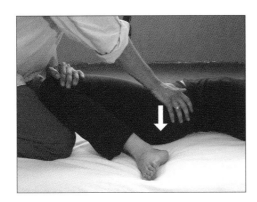

Quadriceps and Iliopsoas Stretch (Step 29)

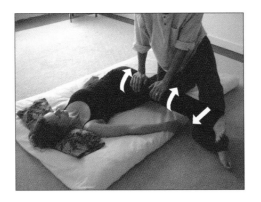

Adduction of Hip (Step 34)

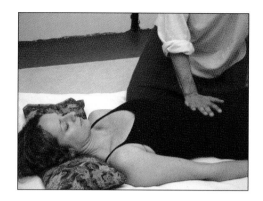

Palm Circles on Stomach (Step 55)

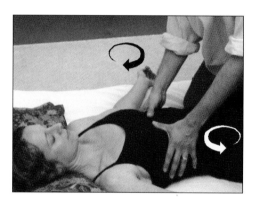

Chest Routine (Steps 51-54)
Reverse the order of the steps so that you are working from the stomach up the chest to the pectoral muscles. Refer back to the acupressure atlas and work with the following point: Torso 13.

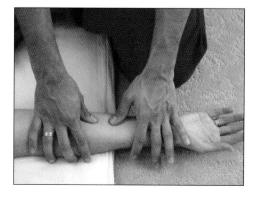

Work Arm Meridians
Continuing with the appropriate side, start and finish this step with a stretch and palm press. Next, thumb press the inner arm lines from the abdomen to the hands. Next, begin again at the shoulder and press the outer arm line. Finish with palm press and stretch.

Refer back to the acupressure atlas and work with the following points: Arms 2, 5, 9, 11, 13, 14, 15, 16, 17, 22, 23.

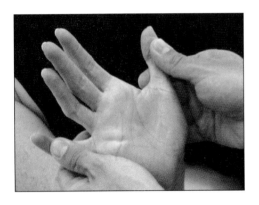

Hand Routine and Acupressure (Steps 36-39)

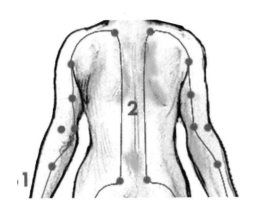

Back Line 2
This step and the next can best be performed with the client in the side-lying position. Walk your thumbs up and down **line 2** on the side you are working with.

Refer back to the acupressure atlas and work with the following points: Back 13, 14, 18, 20, 23.

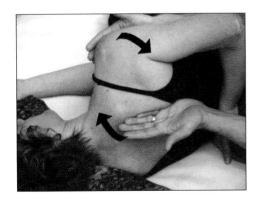

Stretches for Shoulder and Arm (Side variation Steps 6-10)

Having followed the *Kalatharee* from its origin to its terminus, reverse these steps to return to the navel. Then, repeat for the other side.

Therapy Routine for *Sahatsarangsi* and *Tawaree*

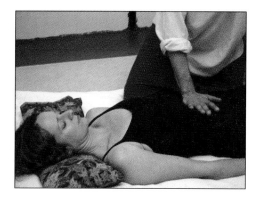

Palm Circles on Stomach (Step 55)
Begin at the navel with a palm circle and palm press.

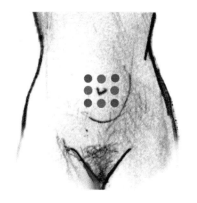

Thumb Press Stomach Points (Step 56)

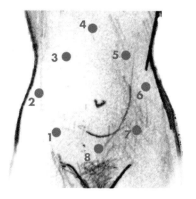

Palm Press Stomach Points (Step 57)
(Use any or all of the three options in Step 57.)

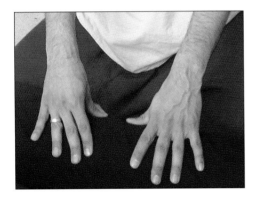

Work Meridians i1 and o2
Beginning with the appropriate side (left for female, right for male), start this step with a stretch and palm press. Next, thumb press line i1 from the abdomen to the foot. Note that because you are working from the navel to the extremities, the direction is reversed from that of the classic routine. Next, begin again at the hip and thumb press line o2 down to the feet. Finish with palm press and stretch. Refer back to the acupressure atlas and work with the following points: Legs 3, 29.

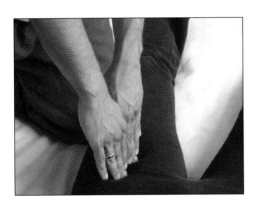

**Femoral Blood Stop and Psoas Press
(Step 16 Advanced Variation, Step 58)**
Press with a bladed hand along the upper thigh and along the iliopsoas muscle.

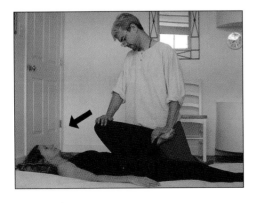

Hip Stretch (Step 25)

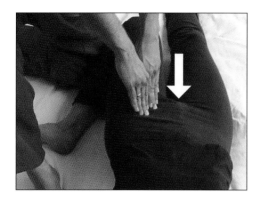

**Quadriceps Stretch and Psoas Press
(Step 29 and Advanced Variation)**

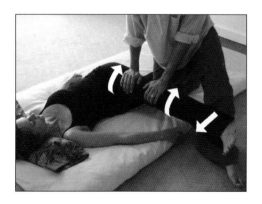

Hip Adduction (Step 34)

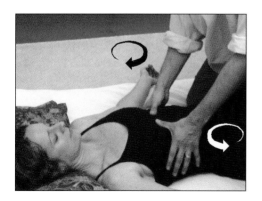

Abdominal Routine (Steps 51-55)
Reverse the order of these steps so that you are working from the lower abdomen up to the pectoral muscles.

Also with thumb presses, follow the course of the Sahatsarangsi or Tawaree meridian up the chest from the abdomen to the neck. Refer back to the acupressure atlas and work with the following point: Torso 12.

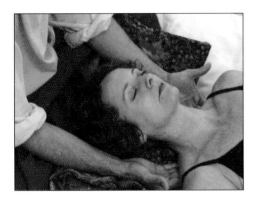

Neck Lines and Acupressure (Steps 101, 103)

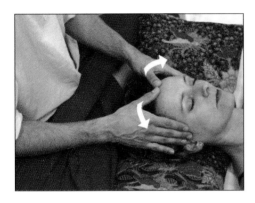

Head and Face Routine (Steps 105-106)

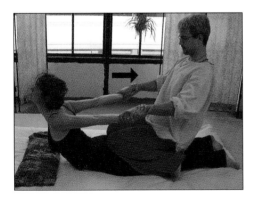

**Back Bends
(Steps 98, 99, and Side-lying Variations)**
Back bends engage the entire front of the body, and activate these meridians.

Having followed the *Sahatsarangsi* or *Tawaree* from its origin to its terminus, reverse these steps to return to the navel. Then, repeat for the other side.

Therapy Routine for *Sumana*

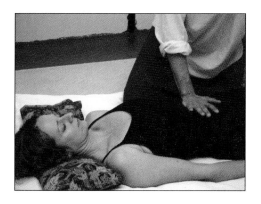

Palm Circles on Stomach (Step 55)
Begin at the navel with a palm circle and palm press.

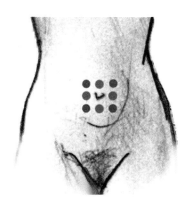

Thumb Press Stomach Points (Step 56)

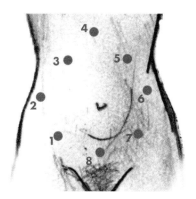

Palm Press Stomach Points (Step 57)
(Use any or all of the three options presented in Step 57.)

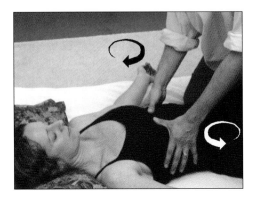

Chest Routine (Steps 51-54)

Reverse the order of these steps so that you are working from the lower abdomen up to the pectoral muscles.

Refer back to the acupressure atlas and work with the following points: Torso 10, 16, 17.

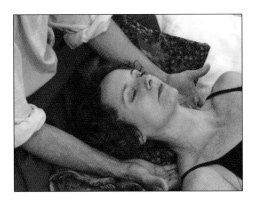

Neck Lines and Trapezius Routine (Steps 101, 103)

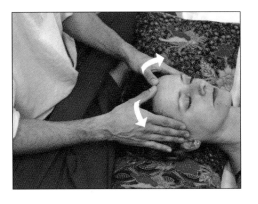

Head and Face Routine (Step 105)

Refer back to the acupressure atlas and work with the following point: Head 8, 16, 17, 19.

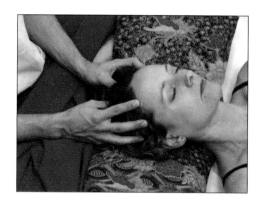

Crown Chakra (Step 106)

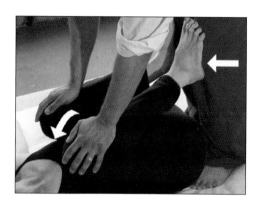

Abdominal Compression (Step 61)

Spinal Twist (Step 28 or 75)

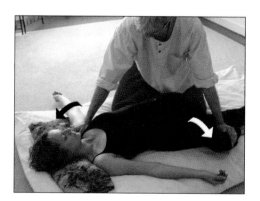

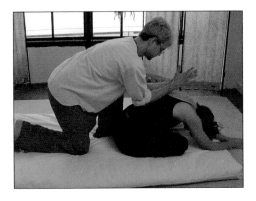

Forward Bends (Steps 65-72)

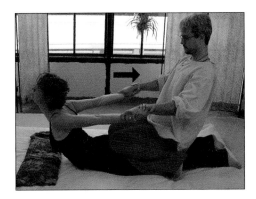

Back Bends
(Steps 98, 99, and Side-lying Variations)
Back bends engage the entire front of the body,
and activate this meridian.

**Having followed the *Sumana* from its origin to its
terminus, reverse these steps to return to the navel.**

Therapy Routine for *Lawusang* and *Ulanga*

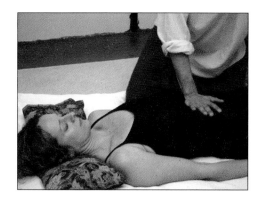

Palm Circles on Stomach (Step 55)
Begin at the navel with a palm circle and palm press.

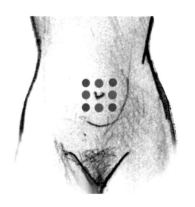

Thumb Press Stomach Points (Step 56)

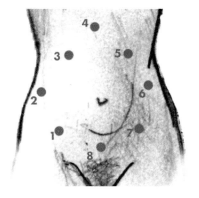

Palm Press Stomach Points (Step 57)
Use any or all of the three options in Step 57.)

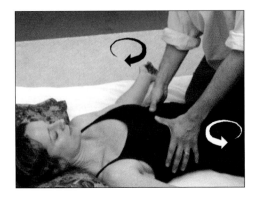

Chest Routine (Steps 51-54)

Reverse the order of these steps so that you are working from the lower abdomen up to the pectoral muscles. For these meridians, you can work on both sides of the body at the same time.

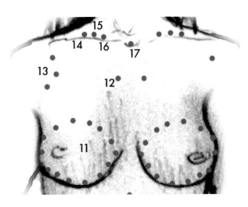

Acupressure on Thoracic Region

Also with thumb presses, follow the line of the *Lawusang* and *Ulanga* meridians from the navel to the neck. (Skipping over the breasts if this is not appropriate.)

Refer back to the acupressure atlas and work with the following points: Torso 11, 12, 14, 15, 16.

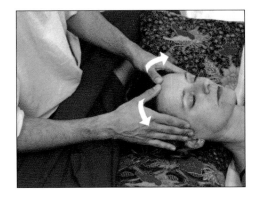

Head and Face Routine (Step 105)

Refer back to the acupressure atlas and work with the following points: Head 5, 12, 13.

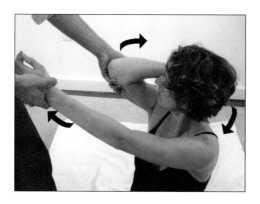

Neck Stretch (Seated Position 7)

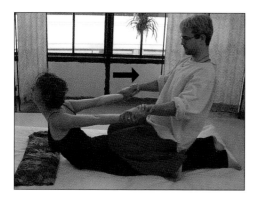

**Back Bends
(Steps 98, 99, and Side-lying Variations)**
Back bends engage the entire front of the body, and activate these meridians.

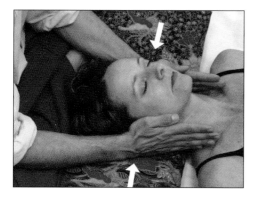

**Crown Chakra and Ear Vacuum
(Steps 106-107)**
The ear vacuum is particularly important for this meridian.

Having followed the *Lawusang-Ulanga* from its origin to its terminus, reverse these steps to return to the navel.

Therapy Routine for *Nantakawat*

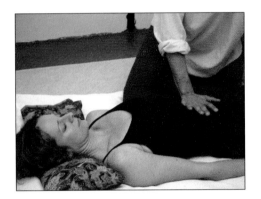

Palm Circles on Stomach (Step 55)
Begin at the navel with a palm circle and palm press.

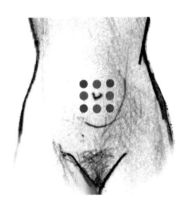

Thumb Press Stomach Points (Step 56)

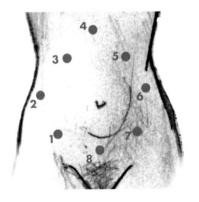

Palm Press Stomach Points (Step 57)
(Use any or all of the three options presented in Step 57.)

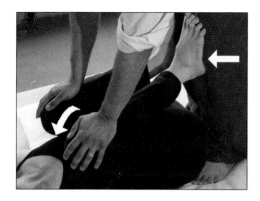

Gentle Back Stretch with Abdominal Compression (Step 61)

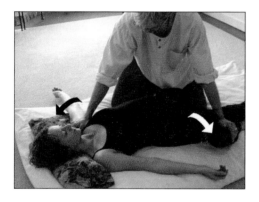

Spinal Twist (Step 28)
Repeat for both sides.

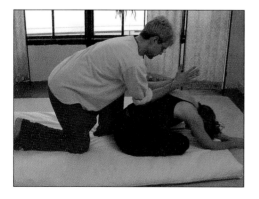

Forward Bends (Steps 65-72)
Forward bends help by compressing the abdomen and stretching the lower back. If your client wishes to perform back bends as well, this is beneficial, however you should place the client in the side-lying position so as not to put pressure on the abdominal region.

Finish by repeating abdominal steps.

Therapy Routine for *Kitcha*

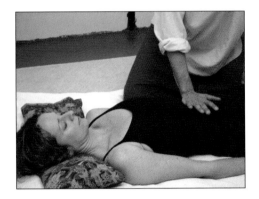

Palm Circles on Stomach (Step 55)
Begin at the navel with a palm circle and palm press.

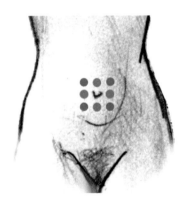

Thumb Press Stomach Points (Step 56)

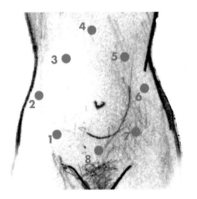

Palm Press Stomach Points (Step 57)
(Use any of all of the three options presented in Step 57.)

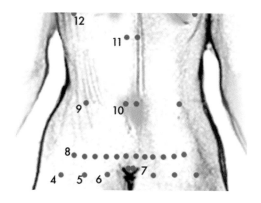

Acupressure for Lower Back
Refer back to the acupressure atlas and work with the following points: Back 8, 9, 10, 11.

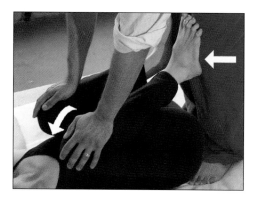

Gentle Back Stretch with Abdominal Compression (Step 61)

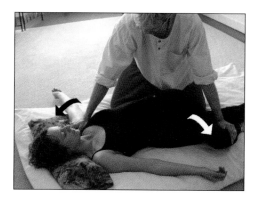

Spinal Twist (Step 28)
Repeat for both sides.

Finish by repeating abdominal steps.

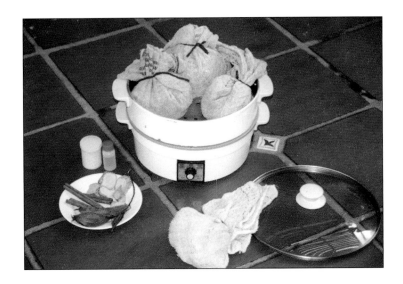

Chapter 9
Thai Herbs and Massage

Thai Herbs

Herbs are an everyday part of Thai life, and are used in traditional Thai healing for their rejuvenating and balancing effects on the body, mind, and energy. In my book, *A Thai Herbal: Traditional Recipes for Health and Harmony*, I discuss the holistic world-view of the Thai healer and the role of herbs in traditional Thai medicine. In fact, along with massage and spiritual practice, herbalism is one of the three main branches of Thai medicine.

There is significant overlap between Thai herbalism and massage, as I will discuss in this chapter, and no Thai massage clinic in Thailand will go without some of the essentials of herbal healing.

Herbal Compress Massage

One of the most interesting ways in which these two disciplines dovetail is in the herbal compress massage known as *Luk Pra Kob*. This is a unique form of massage which is also practiced mainly in spas in Thai beach-side resorts, and which is now becoming increasingly popular in the West. An herbal massage incorporates heated herbal compresses into the traditional Thai massage with which you are already familiar. Herbal compresses are heated in an herbal steamer (shown above), and the warm bundles are applied directly to the skin or through the client's clothing during a massage session.

It is no secret that hot compresses are excel-

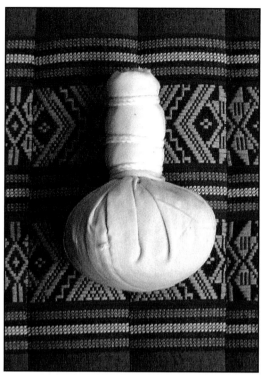

Herbal compress bundle.

lent for stiff, sore, or pulled muscles and ligaments; back pain; arthritis; chronic pain or injury; disorders of the internal organs; skin diseases, migraines, and chronic stress or anxiety. But a hot herbal compress adds to these benefits the healing effects of therapeutic herbs. The blend of traditional Thai herbs used in these compresses has simultaneously a relaxing and invigorating effect on the body and mind, soothing sore and overworked muscles while giving a boost for the body's energy level.

The two blends of herbs discussed in this chapter are the traditional recipe from around the Chiang Mai area, and the traditional recipe of the Wat Po temple in Bangkok. These are not, however, the only recipes used in Thailand. Herbs for the compresses are blended with attention to the therapeutic needs of the individual, such as for arthritis, cold, flu, fever, and other illnesses, and most massage therapists have

Recipes for Herbal Compresses

Lay out three thin muslin or cotton cloths in front of you. Place ingredients on each cloth, and wrap tightly to make a small bundle. Place bundles in the steamer and cook at 250° for 15 to 20 minutes. Remove one by one. Allow to cool sufficiently before using with client. (Test each bundle on your forearm before using.) Apply compresses to client's skin with moderate pressure. When each compress has cooled, place it back in the steamer to re-heat. Compresses may be re-used for up to 2 hours before being discarded. Always use fresh herbs for each session. There are two classic recipes for herbal compresses, although many other variations can be improvised:

Wat Po: The traditional recipe from the Southern lineage in Bangkok. Start with a fist full of cassumunar ginger (*Zingiber cassumunar*) for each compress. Add another handful of lemongrass (*Cymbopogon citratus*) and kaffir lime leaves (*Citrus hystix*) combined. Finish each compress with a liberal sprinkle of camphor crystals (*Cinnamomum camphora*).

Chiang Mai: This recipe is used by many providers in the Chiang Mai area, and is taught by the Shivago lineage. Begin with a handful of Cassumunar ginger. Add a combined handful of kaffir lime leaves and rind, eucalyptus leaves (*Eucalyptus globulus*), and cinnamon leaves (*Cinnamomum zeylanicum*). Finish each compress with a liberal sprinkle of camphor crystals.

Note: Common ginger (*Zingiber officinale*) may be substituted for Cassumunar, but try to avoid other substitutions. Also, essential oils are not suitable for compresses since they tend to dissipate quickly in the steamer. Many of the herbs mentioned above are available at Thai markets, and through my school. (See back of this book for contact information.)

several different favorite recipes they use on a regular basis. (For more information on custom herbal blends for individual clients, please consult *A Thai Herbal*, which discusses this and other aspects of traditional Thai herbalism in detail.)

Herbal compress application is an integral part of Thai "hot therapy" discussed in Chapter 7. Refer back to the diagram of the blocked *sen* line. Note how the patient with blocked energy meridians can benefit from direct pressure to the location of the blockage. While "hot pressure" may be called for in this case, many of these clients will be too sensitive to receive massage or acupressure therapy directly on this location. The herbal compress can be a useful way to apply hot pressure along *sen* lines, acupressure points, and joints that could not otherwise be massaged, and is considered to be as effective a method of delivering hot pressure as acupressure. Simply apply the compress to the site (as hot as the client can stand without

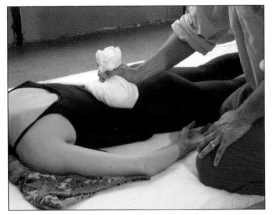

Applying hot herbal compresses.

burning), and press gently with your palm.

Note that often, ill or sensitive clients can have a very relaxing and invigorating experience with herbal compresses, without use of any yogic stretches at all. Hot compresses provide marked relief of symptoms associated with arthritis or other joint stiffness, and help these clients to be able to perform yoga stretches that would otherwise be impossible. I have also had wonderful results when working with clients with fibromyalgia and other chronic pain disorders.

Other Herbs for Compresses

The following herbs are also used in the Thai compress. Experiment with adding these herbs into the traditional recipes on the previous page. (More information on each of these plants is available in *A Thai Herbal*.)

Calamus *(Acorus calamus)*
Cayenne oil *(Capsicum frutescens)*
Cloves *(Syzygium aromaticum)*
Garlic *(Allium sativum)*
Jasmine *(Jasminum officinale, others)*
Lemon Rind *(Citrus limonum)*
Mandarin Orange Rind *(Citrus reticulata)*
Sea Salt *(Sodium chloride)*
Soap Nut *(Sapindus rarak)*
Tamarind *(Tamarindus indica)*
Turmeric *(Curcuma longa)*
Zedoary *(Curcumin zedoaria)*
Zerumbet Ginger *(Zingiber zerumbet)*

Hot compresses can be used in conjunction with Thai massage in several other ways. Many clinics in Thailand use the herbal compresses as a relaxing way to soothe a client's hard-working muscles after the Thai massage work. Typically, this will add on 15-20 minutes to the massage routine. The entire body will be pressed with hot compresses to ease any residual tension in the muscles.

Use of the compress during the course of the massage can be relaxing and also stimulating. Thai therapists can use herbal compresses on the joints in order to soften and loosen the connections between bones and increase mobility before major stretching, while use of the compresses on the abdomen can encourage digestion and stimulate the organs. Apply the hot compresses to the skin directly or through the client's massage clothes, and allow them to warm the client's body, penetrating and dissipating any tension before moving on to deep acupressure work.

Another idea is to use the compresses as heating pillows, as a prop for the client's neck, head, or the backs of the knees. You may also wish to leave compresses at important acupressure points in order to stimulate the energy flow throughout the body. Applying compresses to palms or soles of the feet can also have the same effect. Experiment with different locations on the body, but be sure to avoid the eyes and other areas which may be sensitive.

Hot compress massage is also an excellent option for post-partum clients, who should not be receiving a full Thai massage from a non-specialist. Most parts of the body — including the limbs, hands and feet — can be pressed with herbal compress in order to relax muscles and impart the benefits of the herbs. The stomach and lower abdominal areas should not be pressed, however, so as not to disturb the natural processes taking place. As always, be sure that you have adequate knowledge of the herbs being used, and a full understanding of their potential effects with regards to any medical condition.

The aromatherapy effects of the herbs used in the compresses should not be undervalued. Many of these herbs have a balancing effect on the mind and spirit, and provide clients with a soothing reduction of stress. All of the herbs also possess properties which clear out congestion of the lungs and sinuses, and application of hot compresses to the chest and throat can be a wonderful way to kick a cold.

Another use of herbal compresses that should be mentioned is the application of cold compresses. Cold compresses should be cooked for 25-30 minutes to release the beneficial alkaloids in the herbs, and then frozen or iced. The cold compresses should then be applied to clients with muscle strains, tendon or ligament sprains, contusions, hematomas, and more severe injuries requiring "cold therapy." (See Chapter 7.) Cold compresses help to reduce swelling and pain and can promote dissipation of pooled stagnant energy due to broken *sen* lines. Cold compresses should be applied only to the site of the injury and should be monitored while the practitioner massages other areas of the body.

Herbal Balms and Other Topical Applications

Even if no hot compresses are used, a typical Thai massage in Thailand is often followed by the application of an herbal balm or liniment to soothe and relax the muscles which have been hard at work. Many clinics offer home-made preparations, which may come in varying strengths and aromas. These topical applications have the effect of stimulating circulation to the muscles, which helps to warm and detoxify the body. Also, many of these preparations serve as mild analgesics, which lessen pain or soreness.

Tiger Balm™ is often the most convenient choice in the West, where this product is readily available in drug and vitamin stores. However, the entrepreneurial Thai therapist may also wish to experiment with making his or her own herbal balm, and with this individual in mind, I offer the following recipe. This recipe is for a balm similar to Tiger Balm™, but you may wish to experiment with different essential oils in order to create custom blends. Any relatively aromatic or spicy herb can be used topically to soothe sore muscles. Refer to my book, *A Thai Herbal*, for a complete list of Thai herbs in these categories.

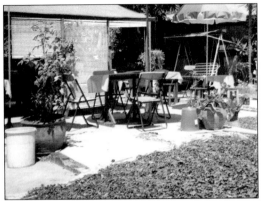

Drying herbs for the sauna at the Traditional Medicine Hospital.

Herbal Sauna or Steam Bath

Every massage clinic worth its salt in Chiang Mai has a sauna or steam bath for clients to use after receiving Thai massage. The purpose of the sauna is to relax the muscles after the intensive massage, but also to release through the pores toxins broken up by the bodywork. Sweating is one of the body's natural purification methods, and the Thais have traditionally used herbs in the sauna to assist in this process. The classic recipe for a Thai sauna is the same as the recipe for the herbal compresses, although many different aromatic herbs may be added to achieve particular purposes or to address particular needs. (See *A Thai Herbal* for more information and recipes for herbal inhalation.)

Home-Made Tiger Balm™

10 drops essential oil of peppermint
10 drops essential oil of eucalyptus
5 drops essential oil of cinnamon
5 drops essential oil of clove
60 ml. extra-virgin olive oil or coconut oil
15 grams beeswax

Heat olive oil and beeswax in a double-boiler over low heat. Stir until wax is melted. Remove from heat. Stir in essential oils, and pour into small glass or metal containers to cool.

Note that commercial Tiger Balm™ is available in several strengths, and that you may adjust the quantities of essential oils in this recipe. This balm may also be made using Vaseline™ or other petroleum jelly as a base for a consistency closer to Tiger Balm™.

The Chiang Mai sauna can range from a tile-walled steam chamber to a simple box made with sheet metal. The steam can be pumped in through a complex system of pipes, or can be delivered simply by placing an herbal steamer with an open lid under the client's seat. Whatever method you use, the Thai herbal sauna is an experience your clients will never forget.

In the sauna or steam bath, essential oils can be used to substitute for difficult to find or expensive Thai herbs. I have also has good results using Thai essential oils in the bathtub for a relaxing soak after a Thai massage session.

Appendices

Endnotes

1. Brun & Schumacher, 34
2. Ratarasarn, 277-78
3. Brust, Thai Traditional Massage
4. Brust, Thai Traditional Massage
5. Zysk, 53-54
6. Apfelbaum, 25-26
7. Frawley 1999, 223-225

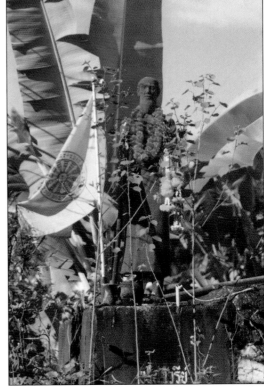

**The Father Doctor at the
Shivagakomarpaj Institute, Chiang Mai**

Sources

Apfelbaum, Ananda. *Thai Massage: Sacred Bodywork*. New York: Avery, 2004

Brust, Harald (Asokananda). *The Art of Thai Traditional Massage*. Bangkok: Editions Duang Kamol, 1990

Brust, Harald (Asokananda). *Thai Traditional Massage for Advanced Practitioners*. Bangkok: Editions Duang Kamol, 1996

Frawley, David. *Yoga and Ayurveda: Self-Healing and Self-Realization*. Twin Lakes, WI: Lotus Press, 1999

Ratarasarn, Somchintana. *The Principles and Concepts of Thai Classical Medicine*. Bangkok: Thai Khadi Research Institute, Thammasat University, 1986

Salguero, C. Pierce. *A Thai Herbal: Recipes for Health and Harmony*. Forres, Scotland: Findhorn Press, 2003

Zysk, Kenneth G. *Asceticism and Healing in Ancient India: Medicine in the Buddhist Monastery*. Delhi: Motilal Banarsidass, 1998

Anatomical Terms Used in this Book
& Anatomy Charts

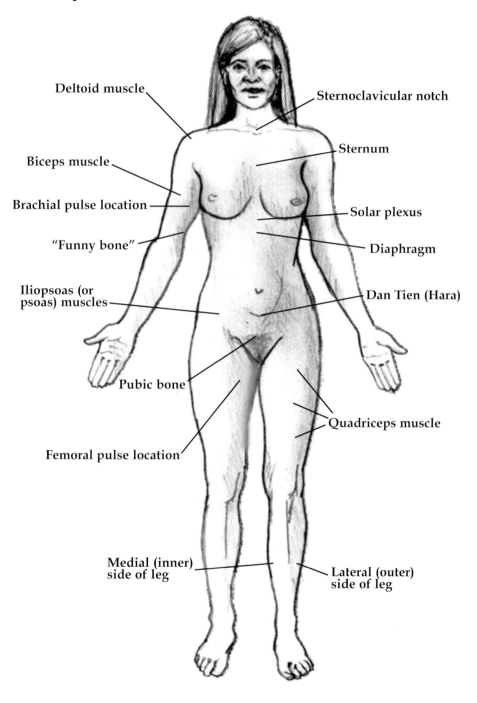

Deltoid muscle

Sternoclavicular notch

Sternum

Biceps muscle

Brachial pulse location

Solar plexus

"Funny bone"

Diaphragm

Iliopsoas (or psoas) muscles

Dan Tien (Hara)

Pubic bone

Quadriceps muscle

Femoral pulse location

Medial (inner) side of leg

Lateral (outer) side of leg

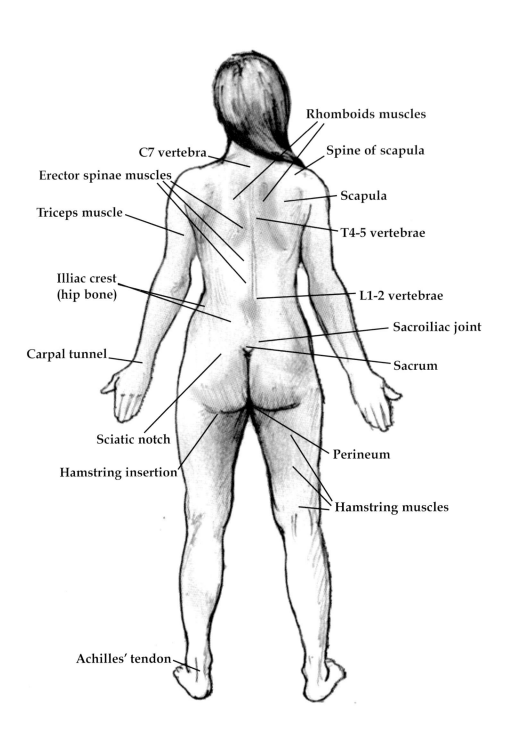

Rhomboids muscles

C7 vertebra

Spine of scapula

Erector spinae muscles

Scapula

Triceps muscle

T4-5 vertebrae

Illiac crest
(hip bone)

L1-2 vertebrae

Sacroiliac joint

Carpal tunnel

Sacrum

Sciatic notch

Perineum

Hamstring insertion

Hamstring muscles

Achilles' tendon

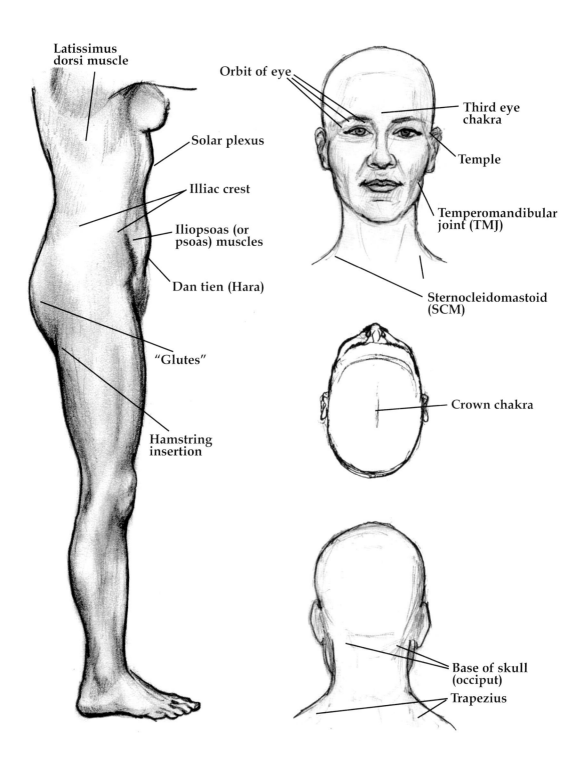

Latissimus
dorsi muscle

Orbit of eye

Third eye
chakra

Solar plexus

Temple

Illiac crest

Temperomandibular
joint (TMJ)

Iliopsoas (or
psoas) muscles

Dan tien (Hara)

Sternocleidomastoid
(SCM)

"Glutes"

Crown chakra

Hamstring
insertion

Base of skull
(occiput)

Trapezius

Where to Study Thai Massage

I am always asked by students and prospective students where the best places to study Thai massage are. My own feeling, as I often tell them, is that anyone hoping to learn Thai massage therapy should seek out the best institutions in their own country to learn the classic routine before traveling to Thailand. I feel that a traveler with a few weeks or months to spend in Thailand is not served by spending this precious time learning the basics in a crowded class of tourists who may or may not take this art form seriously. Most Western students will, moreover, find themselves disappointed by the lack of theoretical teaching at most Thai schools, as well as by the inevitable language barrier that still exists in most places.

On the other hand, the traveler who is already familiar with Thai massage and has a decent background in the theory can travel to Chiang Mai or Bangkok and learn directly from practitioners of this art by receiving, observing, and discussing massage in a less formal setting. There is an older generation of true masters practicing in tucked-away corners of Chiang Mai and Bangkok. These people have neither websites nor international marketing tools, and thus remain relatively unknown to prospective travelers. These are the individuals with whom one can truly see the highest levels of perfection of this art form, and with whom it is a privilege to work. But, it requires that you to travel to Thailand, track them down, and spend the time getting to know them. This, in my view, is the most rewarding way to learn this tradition, and is an experience the traveler will never forget.

Of course, readers who are planning on spending a lengthy period of time in Thailand can ignore all of the above and jump right into a basic class knowing that they will have plenty of time to spend with the masters at a later date. This is the route that I took, and it is entirely possible to

spend several years in Thailand learning the traditional healing arts while supporting one's self by teaching English or by working with non-profit organizations. The benefits of learning in Thailand are many, not least of all the cultural experience and personal connections that can be made.

Studying Thai Massage at Home

Searching for a basic course in Thai massage outside of Thailand can seem like a daunting process. Many schools talk about their lineage, their techniques, and other facets of their teachings in ways that can be confusing and sometimes misleading to beginning students. In reality, most Thai massage schools in the West essentially teach the classic routine introduced in Chapter 4 in their basic course (give or take a few of the steps). When you are looking for a school, keep in mind that the major difference from place to place is not the content but the atmosphere, the cultural knowledge of the teacher, and the attention to safety and proper body mechanics.

When looking at a school, be sure that the teacher studied in Thailand, and didn't simply watch a video or take a weekend seminar somewhere. (Beware: this happens more often than you would think!) Unfortunately, most schools in the West—either in an attempt to appeal to the Western clinical massage setting, or else out of an ignorance of the traditions—have stripped out important cultural elements of traditional Thai massage training. Be sure that the school teaches the history, theory, and culture of Thai healing.

Any serious school will include daily ceremonies addressed to the Father Doctor, and will follow the traditional code of ethics of the Thai healer. This should be your minimum criteria in choosing a school. Also, be sure that the teachers' know to which lineage they belong. As in most Asian arts, in Thai massage, lineage is an important mark of authenticity. In the traditional viewpoint, the teacher who does not know his or her lineage is not worth studying with.

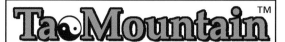

**School of Traditional Thai
Massage & Herbal Medicine**
www.TaoMountain.org   www.Thai-Herbs.com

In the interests of promoting the integrity of Thai traditions and the culture of Thai healing, my organization, Tao Mountain, maintains a website with a large quantity of information and resources about Thai massage and herbal medicine. We maintain a free monthly newsletter to keep the public abreast of interesting developments and topics in the world of Thai medicine, and also provide links to Basic, Advanced, and Teacher Training courses. Our Thai herbs website offers Thai massage related products as well as hard-to-find Thai herbs used for massage compresses. For more information, contact me through the above websites.

Studying Massage in Thailand

The recommendations I make in this section have to be taken with a grain of salt. Thailand is a developing country and the situation there changes drastically over the course of a few years. The traveler seeking to learn Thai massage in the country of its origin will be faced with a quite different reality than when I took my first course in 1997, or when I taught my last course at the Traditional Medicine Hospital in 2000. As the popularity of this modality grows, courses at the best schools are becoming over-crowded. Furthermore, many students are not professional therapists, but rather fun-seeking backpackers, leading to a sometimes boisterous classroom environment. However, I give the following recommendations based on the long-standing respect with which these institutions have been regarded.

Although each of these schools offers an introductory course, each teaches its own particular style of healing, and it is possible to attend all three institutions and have a unique experience at each. Note that there are many other schools and renowned private instructors in Thailand, although the serious student should be aware that these schools are not always reputable. Also note that even at the schools mentioned here, it is not always possible or advisable to register in advance. The best course of action for any student is usually to travel to Chiang Mai or Bangkok without a plan, gauge for yourself the lie of the land, and decide in person the best places to study.

Shivagakomarpaj Institute Traditional Medicine Hospital

**78/1 Wuolai Rd., Chiang Mai 50100
www.thaimassageschool.ac.th**

Chiang Mai's Foundation of Shivagakomarpaj Traditional Medicine Hospital is, according to many, Thailand's premier massage school. Their course features a decent introduction to the theory and practice of Thai medicine (when the theory teacher is in residence, that is). The Traditional Medicine Hospital's ten-day course is one of the best offered on this subject for beginners and professionals alike, although recently classes have been unfortunately over-crowded. Upon completion of ten days, a certification exam is given (although virtually no Thai certificates are recognized in Western countries). Graduates of the foundation are on occasion able to continue their education by volunteering as "interns" with subsequent courses. Readers of this book will find that the Traditional Medicine Hospital's curriculum follows closely the material presented in these pages. This is because I both learned and taught at this institute, and consider it to be my primary influence.

Lek Chaiya's
Nerve Touch Massage

25 Rajadamnoen Rd., Muang Chiang Mai 50200
www.NerveTouch.com

Perhaps the best short course on traditional massage can be found at Lek Chaiya Massage, in downtown Chiang Mai. As a former director of the prestigious Association of Northern Herbs, and with over 40 years of massage experience, "Mama" Lek has impeccable credentials and a well-respected unique style. Although she does not speak much English, Lek Chaiya has several employees who serve as both assistant teachers and translators. Students can take three- to five-day courses. Instruction is both by demonstration and hands-on practice, and covers topics from acupressure points and energy meridians to herbal compresses and other therapies. Some of the advanced variations in this book are based on Mama Lek's techniques, which are closer to the Southern style lineage.

Mama Lek's son, Tananan "Maew" Willson, runs a medicinal tea bar below her studio with an extensive menu of Thailand's favorite herbal remedies. For any who are interested in pursuing the study of traditional Thai massage or herbal medicine from a true master, I could not recommend Lek Chaiya's school more highly.

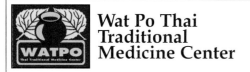

Wat Po Thai Traditional Medicine Center

Sanamachai Rd., Bangkok 10200
www.watpo.com

Wat Po (or Wat Pho) is a well-known tourist temple in Bangkok which has for well over a century been the center of gravity for the serious study of Thai massage and herbal medicine. This is the headquarters of the

Southern style lineage, and is recognized, along with the Traditional Medicine Hospital, as one of the top two schools in the country. Wat Po offers 30-hour courses, which are taken 3 hours per day over 10 days. It offers both a basic and an advanced therapeutic course. Wat Po is also, to my knowledge, the only place where it is possible to study Thai herbal medicine formally. Although the language barrier is formidable, it is possible to take a 1-3 year course in traditional Thai medicine.

More Options

There are many more locations to study and receive massage than I can possibly mention here, and new facilities are constantly popping up. The following are some well-known schools in and around Chiang Mai. Even if you do not study at all of these places, the traveler to Thailand should make a point of at least receiving a massage at these facilities to get a sense of the different styles of each.

Baan Nit (Soi 2, Th. Chaiyaphum, Chiang Mai)
One of the most interesting and colorful experiences I had in my Thai massage education was learning with Mama Nit. A very unstructured, informal, and intuitive learning environment, but a real treat to work with such a powerful energy worker. One-on-one instruction is usually possible, and terms are negotiable.

Pichet Boonthume
(3/3 M. 5 T. Bahn Vehn A., Hang Dong)
Another well-known character in Chiang Mai's Thai massage elite. A teacher with a very unique style, learning with Pichet is definitely worth the experience.

Sunshine Network Institute
(www.asokananda.com)
Asokananda pioneered the study of Thai Massage in the 1980s, and wrote the first books on the subject in any European language. Although his practice of Thai

Massage is heavily influenced by Indian ideas, his school in Chiang Mai has one of the more well-known programs of study.

Thai Massage School of Chiang Mai
(www.1thaimassage.com)
A new school, still unproven, but one which promises high-quality programs for very serious students. Government-accredited 300, 500 and 600 hour programs are taught in English at two locations in Chiang Mai. Teacher certification is also available, as are educational visas for long-term stays (up to 1 year).

Further Reading

In addition to the sources cited at the end of this book, I recommend the following titles for further reading. All of these are in print and readily available as of the time of this writing.

Thai Medicine and Herbal Traditions
Salguero, C. Pierce. *A Thai Herbal: Recipes for Health and Harmony*. Forres, Scotland: Findhorn Press, 2001 — This book is the only English-language guide to the traditional herbal medicine of Thailand. An introduction to Thai medical theory, including Four Element diagnosis is presented, with particular emphasis on diet, natural health and beauty products, and herbal tonics. A chapter on herbal compresses details several recipes, and the compendium of over 150 herbs allows for detailed comparison of medicinal properties. Indexes in English, Thai, and Latin, as well as by ailment, action, and taste.

Anatomy and Physiology
Calais-Germain, Blandine. *Anatomy of Movement*. Seattle: Eastland Press, 1993. – In my opinion, this is the best introduction to anatomy and how it relates to the movement of the body. I consider it to be required reading for my advanced students, and feel it would be beneficial for any body worker, yoga instructor, or massage therapist.

Coulter, H. David. *Anatomy of Hatha Yoga: A Manual for Students, Teachers, and Practitioners*. Honesdale, PA: Body and Breath, Inc., 2001 — An impressive and complete guide to the anatomy and physiology of the practice of yoga. This is a very thick and complex book, and may not be appropriate for the beginner. However, it is essential to the serious practice of hatha yoga or of Thai massage. Chapter 1 is particularly interesting.

Yoga
Iyengar, B.K.S. *Light on Yoga: Revised Edition*. New York: Schocken Books, 1979 — As it states on the front cover of my edition of this book, this is "the Bible of modern yoga by the world's foremost teacher." This is a lighter read than Coulter's book, but is still geared towards the fairly advanced practitioner of hatha yoga. Even so, I consider it indispensible for the Thai therapist.

Silva, Mira and Shyam Mehta. *Yoga the Iyengar Way: The New Definitive Illustrated Guide*. New York: Alfred A. Knopf, 2003 — A highly readable and attractive pictorial guide to the practice of hatha yoga. This is a great book for beginning students of yoga and Thai massage. The postures are explained in detail, with detailed points of alignment.

Ayurvedic Medicine

Frawley, David, et al. *Ayurveda and Marma Therapy: Energy Points in Yogic Healing.* Twin Lakes, WI: Lotus Press, 2003 — A great book for comparison between Ayurvedic and Thai acupressure therapy. Frawley is readable and informative.

Frawley, David. *Yoga and Ayurveda: Self-Healing and Self-Realization.* Twin Lakes, WI: Lotus Press, 1999 — Another readable book useful for comparison. Frawley draws connections between Ayurvedic principles such as *doshas* and the practices of hatha yoga.

Chinese Medicine

Li, Ding. *Acupuncture: Meridian Theory and Acupuncture Points.* Beijing: Foreign Language Press, 1991 — A useful point of comparison between Chinese and Thai acu-points.

Travel to Thailand

Cummings, Joe, et al. *Thailand: 10th Edition.* Melbourne: Lonely Planet Publications, 2003 — This is the pre-eminent guidebook for budget travel to Thailand, but is also a great read. The Lonely Planet series is known for being a reliable and interesting source of cultural information as well as for covering all of the details you need to know to visit.

O'Reilly, James and Larry Habegger, eds. *Thailand, True Stories.* San Francisco: Traveler's Tales, Inc., 2002 — This is a fun little book which will give the reader a glimpse into Thai culture and the life of the Western traveler in this colorful country. Each chapter is a separate vignette on some aspect of Thailand. Some stories will make you laugh, some will shatter your illusions, but all will entertain.

Buddhism

Kornfield, Jack. *Living Dharma: Teachings of Twelve Buddhist Masters.* Boston: Shambhala, 1996 — Buddhism in Southeast Asia has very little to do with the Tibetan and Zen traditions more familiar in the West. This book is a wonderful introduction to twelve Buddhist teachers, half of whom were native to Thailand. Kornfield, a well-known meditation teacher himself, covers the breadth of teaching styles and meditation techniques taught in Theravada Buddhism. This is a great place to start for those interested in pursuing Thai Buddhism and/or Vipassana meditation.

Images of Thailand

Jotisalikorn, Chami. *Thai Spa Book: The Natural Asian Way to Health and Beauty.* Hong Kong: Periplus Editions, 2002. — This is a beautiful book with excellent photos. It presents a very attractive (although not extensive) guide to some Thai beauty and herbal treatments. A great gift or a coffee-table book for your massage clinic.

Warren, William and Luca Invernizzi. *Thailand: The Golden Kingdom.* Hong Kong: Periplus Editions, 1999. — The same photographer as the above book. Provides excellent views of Thailand's beauty. Another nice gift or coffee-table book.

Index

Abdomen   60, 69, 87, 94, 98, 110, 113,
                    123, 133–134, 139, 164, 170, 184

Abdominal Muscles   54, 65

Abdominal Pain   59, 95, 188

Acid Reflux   188

Acupressure   10, 17, 21, 24, 192,
                    194, 206, 207, 236, 237

Acupressure Points   4, 6, 22, 26, 179, 207

Acupuncture   191, 194

Acute Injuries   38, 192

Age   14

Aggression   205

Ajahn Sintorn   7, 9, 10

Amulets   9

Analgesics   237

Anatomy   viii, 4, 6, 30, 177

Angina   188

Ankle   44–45, 54, 60, 69,
                    73, 85, 98, 122, 139

Anxiety   17, 97, 100, 104,
                    108, 166, 188, 205, 235

Appendicitis   188, 195

Arches Of Feet   54

Architecture   11

Ardha Matsyendrasana   115

Ardha Salabhasana   137

Arm   76, 188

Aromatherapy   14, 237

Arthritis   4, 18, 43, 188, 235, 236

Asthma   69, 97, 100, 115, 133, 166, 168, 188, 195

Astrologers   5

Atmosphere   13

Aura   29

Ayurveda   3–7, 9, 194, 203, 204

Ayutthia   5

Baan Nit   246

Babies   17

Back   65, 94, 98, 100, 110, 113, 117, 123, 133,
                    134, 137, 139, 164, 168, 169

Back Pain   17–18, 37, 61, 65, 67, 72, 73,
                    74, 115, 166, 188, 195, 235

Baddha Konasana   107

Balm   237

Bangkok   6, 7, 8, 10, 235, 244, 245, 246

Baths   193, 238

Bell's Palsy   188

Bhujangasana   133, 134

Bipolar Disorder   188

Blocked Energy, Blocked Sen Line   178–179,
                                         193, 194

Blood Pressure   54, 188

Blood Stop   52, 53, 82, 89, 193

Body Mechanics   22, 37

Bone Injuries   192

Brachial Plexus/Pulse   82

Breast Ailments   186, 188, 195

Breath   14, 35–36, 40

Breathing Difficulty   188, 195

Broken Sen Line   178–179, 193, 237

Bronchitis   188

Buddha   10, 11

Buddhism   4, 5, 8, 9, 10, 29

Buddhist Temples (See Also Wat Po,
Wat Phra Kaew)   vii

"Butterfly Palm Press"   23

Buttocks   133, 134, 137

Calamus   236

Calves   54, 61, 72, 97, 100, 122, 137

Camphor Crystals   235

Cardiac Disorders   52, 188

Cassumunar Ginger   235

"Cat Paws"   23

Cataracts   188

Cayenne Oil   236

Ceiling Rope   14, 27

Chakras   22, 185

Chest   54, 60, 73, 74, 85, 98, 100, 110, 123, 133,
                    134, 139, 164, 166, 170, 182, 184

Chest Pain   188

Chi   29

Chiang Mai   viii, 7, 8, 9, 10, 178, 189, 235,
                    244, 245, 246, 247

Children	17
Chill	188
Chin	144
China	vii, 5, 10, 194, 203
Chinese Medicine	178
Chinese Meridians	177
Chiropractic	43, 160
Chronic Condition	17, 192, 206
Chronic Joint Stiffness (See Arthritis)	
Chronic Pain	18, 235, 236
Cinnamon Leaves	235
Blood Circulation	4, 22, 17, 28
Classic Thai Massage Routine	21, 29–30, 37, 39, 179, 204
Clavicles	87, 140, 141
Client Interviews/Profile Form	14–15
Client Release Form	14, 16
Clothing	14
Cloves	236
Code Of Ethics	7, 8, 244
Cold	188, 235, 237
Cold Compresses	237
Cold Therapy	192, 193, 204
Colon	90, 93, 188
Compassionate	11
Compresses	193
Constipation	188, 195
Contraindications	14
Contusions	237
Cough	188, 195
Cramps	188
Crown Chakra	140, 145
Damaged Tissue	4
Dance	36
Deep Tissue Massage	4
Deltoid Muscles	129
Depression	59, 95, 97, 100, 104, 166, 168, 188
Detoxification	4, 237
Dhanurasana	123, 137
Diagnosis	6, 203–204
Diaphragm	188
Diarrhea	61, 72, 73, 74, 97, 100, 115, 168, 188
Digestion	59, 69, 95, 97, 113, 115, 166, 236
Dizziness	188, 195
Doshas	10, 204, 205
Dull Pain	193
Dwi Pada Sirsasana	103
Ear	141, 145, 186, 188, 195
Eka Pada Rajakapotasana	60, 98
Elbow	79
Elbow Press	26, 29, 192–193
Elderly Individuals	17
Elimination	59, 95
Emotions	19, 204
Energy	4, 10, 19, 20, 29, 37, 40, 179, 185, 191, 192, 203, 204, 234
Energy Flow	19, 29, 178, 237
Energy Imbalance	19, 20, 178
Energy Meridians (See Sen)	
Energy–Work	4
Epilepsy	188
Erectile Dysfunction	188, 195
Essential Oils	237, 238
Eucalyptus Leaves	235
Excretion Organs	187
Exhaustion	19
Exorcisms	9
Eyes	184, 188, 195
Face	140, 161
Facial Pain	195
Facial Paralysis	188
Fainting	195
Father Doctor Shivago (See Shivago)	
Fatigue	4, 168, 188, 195, 205
Fear	205
Femoral Artery/Pulse	52
Fertility	187
Fever	188, 195, 235
Fibromyalgia	18, 236
Finger Circles	25, 29
Finger Pain	188

Finger Press	25, 29	Hiccups	195
Five Precepts	8	High Blood Pressure	52, 61, 65, 69, 72, 91,
Flexibility	4, 17, 18, 29		100, 103–104, 110, 113, 123,
Flu	235		137, 139, 164, 168, 170, 195
Foot	41–42, 65, 117, 139, 188	Hill–Tribe Regions	7
Foot Press	27, 29, 171, 173, 174, 192	Hip	18, 54, 58, 59, 60, 61, 64, 72,
Forearm Roll/Press	26, 29		74, 85, 103, 107, 115, 125, 131, 150
Forehead	144	Hip Flexors	60, 69, 94, 98, 110,
Four Elements	203, 204, 205		113, 123, 137, 139, 164, 170
Gall Bladder	188	Hip Pain	195
Garlic	236	Holistic	5, 234
Gastrointestinal Ailments	18, 188, 195	Hot Compress Massage	18, 192, 234–37
Ginger	235	Hot Compresses	18
Glaucoma	188	Hot Pressure	193, 236
Glutes	126	Hot Therapy	193, 204, 236
Gomukhasana	85, 131	Ice Packs	193
Graduation Ceremonies	11	Ida Nadi	177
Gravity	37	Iliopsoas	36, 70
Groin	54, 60, 61, 72, 97, 98, 103, 107, 109	Imbalance	204
Gum Disease	188	Immune System	4
Guru	10	Inability To Commit	205
Halasana	100	Incantations	9
Hamstring	61, 63, 72, 96,	Incontinence	188
	97, 100, 137, 149	India	vii, 4, 5, 35
Hand	76, 188	Indigenous Thai Medicine	5
Hatha Yoga	6, 9	Indigestion	188, 195
Head	140	Infants	14
Headache	54, 61, 72, 73, 74, 94, 100,	Infertility	188, 195
	104, 110, 113, 123, 133, 134, 137,	Initiation Ceremonies	11
	139, 164, 166, 168, 188, 194, 195	Injury	4, 192, 206, 235
Hearing Loss	188	Inner Thigh	60
Heart	17, 65, 108, 182, 195	Insomnia	19, 100, 113,
Heart Trouble	52, 91, 73, 103, 104, 139, 168,		166, 168, 188, 195
	170, 188	Intake Questionnaire	14
Heel Pain	195	Intercostal Spaces	88, 129
Heel Press	27, 29, 171, 193	Internal Organs	235
Hematomas	237	Interviewing	14
Herbal Balms	237	Intestinal Disease	188
Herbal Compress Massage	17, 234–237	Intracostal Muscles	113
Herbal Compresses	37, 192, 234–237	Iris	203
Herbal Manuscripts	5, 6	Islam	5
Herbalism/Herbalists	10, 204, 234, 246	Itha	177, 180, 182, 188, 189,
Hernia	59, 91, 95, 188		194, 204, 205, 206, 207, 208

Iyengar   35, 40
Janu Sirsasana   97
Jap Sen   191
Jasmine   236
Jaundice   188
Jaw   186, 188
Jealousy   205
Jivaka Komarabaccha   9
Joint Mobilization   17, 22
Joint Pain   37
Joint Stiffness   236
Joints   4, 17
Kaffir Lime Leaves   235
Kalatharee   178, 182, 188,
                                  189, 205, 207, 213
Kapha   204, 205
Karna Pidasana   100
Kidney   93
Kidney Ailments   18, 195
King Asoka   5
Kitcha   187, 188, 189, 205, 207, 232
Kitchana   187
Knee   54, 60, 61, 69, 72, 73, 97,
                              98, 103, 107, 123, 188, 195
Knee Press   27, 29, 171, 192–193
Knuckles   43, 78
Lactation   188
Latissimus Dorsi Muscles ("Lats")   129
Lawusang   186, 188, 189, 205, 207, 227
Leg   54, 65, 73, 74, 139
Leg Pain   188, 195
Lek Chaiya   246
Lemon Rind   236
Lemongrass   235
Lethargy   19, 188, 205
Liability Insurance   14
Liability Release Form   16
Licensing   8
Ligaments   4, 235, 237
Lineage   244
Liniment   14, 237
Liver   188, 195

Low Blood Pressure   74, 103, 110, 123,
                                  137, 139, 164, 170
Low Energy   17
Lower Back   59, 60, 69, 95,
                                  107, 109, 134, 137
Lower Gastrointestinal Disorder   18
Luk Pra Kob (see Herbal Compress Massage)
Lungs   188, 195, 237
Lymph   4, 22, 90, 129
Magicians   5
"Mama" Lek   246
Mandarin Orange Rind   236
Marmas   177, 194
Massage Compresses   245
Massage Mat   13
Matsyasana   113
Mattress   13
Medicinal Herbs   9
Meditation   10, 20, 36
Menstrual Discomfort   61, 65, 72, 97, 107,
                                  108, 115, 166, 195
Menstruation   17, 18, 168, 189, 195
Meridians (See Sen)
Metta   11, 12, 18, 19, 40, 146
Migraines   235
Mobility   4
Monasteries   9, 10
Monks   7
Motion Sickness   195
Mouth   186, 195
Muscle Knots   193
Muscle Strain   35, 192, 237
Muscle Tone   4
Music   14
Mythology   vii
Nadis   177
Nantakawat   187, 188, 189, 205, 207
Nasal Congestion   189
Natarajasana   139
Nauli Kriya   91
Nausea   189, 195
Neck   60, 73, 85, 94, 98, 100, 110, 113, 115,
                  123, 131, 133, 134, 137, 139, 140, 141,

142, 159, 160, 161, 164, 166, 168, 170

Neck Pain 189, 195

Negative Energy 19

Nerve Pain 192

Nervousness 205

Northern Lineage/Style 7, 36, 177–178, 189, 190

Numbness 192, 193

Obesity 18, 148, 205

Obsession 205

Offering 11

Opening Prayer 40

Oral Infection 189

Oral Tradition viii, 5

Organs 4, 91, 177, 179, 193

Osteoporosis 65, 73

Ovaries 187, 189

Over–Sexual 205

Pada Hastasana 104

Pain 17–18, 29, 192

Palang Sak 29

Pali 5, 9, 10

Palm Circles 23, 29

Palm Press 23, 29

Palm–Leaf Medical Scriptures 5

Paralysis 189, 192, 193

Parivrtta Trikonasana 74

Paschimottanasana 108

Patthaya 8

Pavana Muktasana 59, 95

Pawanmuktasana 43

Pectoral Muscles 87, 140

Peptic Ulcer 189

Perineum 187

Physicians 5

Physics 17, 37

Physiology 4, 204

Pichet Boonthume 246

Pillows 13

Pingala 177, 180, 182, 188, 189, 194, 204, 205, 206, 207, 208

Pitta 204, 205

Pittakun 187

Plantar Fasciitis 43

PMS (See Menstrual Discomfort)

Poor Balance 139

Post–Partum 18, 91, 237

Prana/Pranic Sheath 29

Prayer 12, 40

Pregnancy 17, 59, 91, 100, 123, 133, 134, 137, 148, 168, 170

Pressure 35, 192

Props 13, 17, 237

Prostate 168, 187, 189

Prostitution 8

Psoas 136, 154

Psychological Health 182, 189, 195, 204, 205

Pulled Muscles 35, 235

Pulse 203

Qi Gong 20

Quadriceps 60–61, 68–69, 72, 85, 94, 98, 110, 123, 136, 137, 139, 154, 164, 170

Reflexology 4, 194

Reiki viii

Release Form 14, 16

Religious Practice 11

Repetitive Stress Injuries 37

Reproductive System Ailments 189, 195

Respiratory Ailments 18, 189, 195

Rheumatic Heart Disease 189

Rhomboids 131–132, 151, 156, 174

Rhythm 14, 36

Rigidity 205

Royal Medical Tradition 5–6, 8, 11

Rural Medical Tradition 5, 7, 9

Sacroiliac Joints 18, 67, 195

Sacrum 126

Safety 13, 14

Sahatsarangsi 184, 188, 189, 205, 207, 219

Salabhasana 170

Salamba Sarvangasana 168

Sanskrit 10, 29

Sauna 193, 238

Savasana 40

Scalp 145

Schizophrenia 189

Sciatica 61, 65, 72, 73, 107, 115, 133, 134, 195

Sea Salt 236

Sen 4, 6, 7, 19, 21, 22, 24, 29, 30, 81, 177–90, 191–94, 203–07, 236–237

Sen Segments In Arms 33

Sen Segments In Head And Neck 30

Sen Segments In Legs 31

Sen Segments In The Back 34

Septum 189

Setu Bandha Sarvangasan 166

Sex Drive, Lack Of 189, 195

Sex Industry 8

Sexual Dysfunction 189

Sexual Function 187

Shamans 5, 9–10

Shava Udarakarshanasana 67

Shiatsu viii, 4, 13

Shivagakomarpaj Lineage 7

Shivagakomarpaj Traditional Medicine Hospital viii, 7, 8, 9, 10, 11, 178, 238, 245

Shivago 8, 9, 10, 11, 12, 40, 244

Shock 189

Shoulder 54, 73, 79, 85, 100, 110, 115, 123, 130, 131, 133–134, 139, 152, 164, 166, 168, 170, 189, 195

Siam vii

Sikhinee 187

Sinuses 180, 195, 237

Sinusitis 100, 166, 168, 189

Sirshapada Bhumi Sparshasana 94

Skin Diseases 235

Soap Nut 236

Sore Throat 189, 195

Sore Muscles 193, 235

Southern Lineage 7, 36, 39, 128, 177, 189–190, 235, 246

Spinal Injury 67, 74, 100, 115

Spinal Twist 66, 114

Spine 59, 67, 73, 74, 94, 95, 100, 109, 110, 113, 115, 123, 133, 134, 137, 139, 164, 166, 168, 170

Spiritual Balance 182

Spiritual Practice 11, 20

Sports 4

Sprains 4

Stagnated Energy 193, 205

Steam Bath 238

Sternum 88

Stiffness 18, 193, 235

Stomachache 189, 195

Stone Tablets 6, 7

Strains 4

Stress *(See Also Anxiety)* 17, 97, 100, 108, 166, 168, 189, 195, 205, 235, 237

Stretching 21

Sukumand 187

Sumana 177, 185, 188, 189, 205, 207, 223

Sunshine Network Institute 246

Supta Padangushtasana 61, 72

Supta Virasana 69

Sushumna Nadi 177, 185

Swedish Massage viii

Swelling 193

Symptoms 14, 18, 203, 204

Tai Chi 20, 36

Tamarind 236

Tao Mountain School Of Thai Massage And Herbal Medicine 245

Tawaree 184, 188, 189, 205, 207, 219

Teeth 186

Temples 9, 10

Tendons 192, 237

Tendonitis 193

Tension *(See Stress, Anxiety)*

Testes 187

Testicular Disease 189

Thai Chop 28

Thai Fist 28

Thai Massage Schools 244–247

Therapeutic Massage 30, 38

Therapeutic Thai Massage Routine 18, 204, 206, 207

Theravada Buddhism 5, 10

Thigh 73, 98, 109